Praeger Handbook of Sports Medicine and Athlete Health

Praeger Handbook of Sports Medicine and Athlete Health

Volume 3
Psychological Perspectives

Ruben J. Echemendia, PhD, Volume Editor
Claude T. Moorman III, MD, Editor-in-Chief

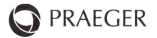 PRAEGER

AN IMPRINT OF ABC-CLIO, LLC
Santa Barbara, California • Denver, Colorado • Oxford, England

Library of Congress Cataloging-in-Publication Data

Praeger handbook of sports medicine and athlete health / Claude T. Moorman III, editor-in-chief.
    p. ; cm.
  Other title: Handbook of sports medicine and athlete health
  Includes bibliographical references and index.
  ISBN 978–0–313–35640–7 (hard paper (set) : alk. paper) — ISBN 978–0–313–35641–4 (ebook (set))
1. Sports medicine—Handbooks, manuals, etc. 2. Athletes—Health and hygiene—Handbooks, manuals, etc. I. Moorman, Claude T. II. Title: Handbook of sports medicine and athlete health.
[DNLM: 1. Sports Medicine. 2. Athletic Injuries. 3. Sports—psychology. QT 261 P897 2011]
RC1211.P73   2011
617.1′027—dc22   2010023432

ISBN: 978–0–313–35640–7
EISBN: 978–0–313–35641–4

15 14 13 12 11   1 2 3 4 5

This book is also available on the World Wide Web as an eBook.
Visit www.abc-clio.com for details.

Praeger
An Imprint of ABC-CLIO, LLC

ABC-CLIO, LLC
130 Cremona Drive, P.O. Box 1911
Santa Barbara, California 93116-1911

This book is printed on acid-free paper ∞

Manufactured in the United States of America

Contents

Preface

Ruben J. Echemendia

Sports have been an important aspect of the human experience since the time of recorded history. It has been observed that sports play a critical role in healthy human development as well as cultural development. Competition is an integral part of human nature, and sports allow for an appropriate channeling of competitive urges and drives. People of all cultures engage in sports activities, and the variety of sports that exists is as diverse as the cultures of the people that engage in those sports. The modern Olympic games are an example of the ubiquitous presence of sports globally and the important role that sports play not only as a vehicle for exercise and fitness but also as a means for diplomacy. Sports also allow for the expression of the peak levels of performance that can be reached through skill, perseverance, dedication, and motivation.

Psychology as a discipline has deep historical roots and a broad reach. Given the centrality of sports in the human experience and the important role that psychology has played in understanding human behavior, it is not surprising that the two have come together in the form of sports psychology—a science that is based on understanding and modifying human behavior in the context of sport and exercise. The discipline of sports psychology is perhaps as varied as the sports that it covers, given that sports psychology is actually an amalgam of psychology, sports and exercise science, anthropology, sociology, and motor learning, to name but a few. In view of the complexity and diversity of sports psychology, it is beyond the scope of this volume to provide an exhaustive review of the scientific literature. Rather than being exhaustive, this volume seeks to acquaint the reader with key aspects of sports psychology by selectively sampling traditional and contemporary areas of inquiry and intervention. Consistent with the other volumes in this set, the chapters that follow will not provide extensive or encyclopedic reference lists. Instead, these chapters begin with the assumption that the reader is new to the scientific study of sports psychology and is seeking a broad introduction to the area. The goal of these chapters, then, is to whet the reader's appetite to engage in further reading and more in-depth study of those areas that are personally appealing.

The volume begins with a historical overview of sports psychology that traces the historical underpinnings of the discipline, the factors that shaped various lines of inquiry, the emergence of governance bodies, the internal tensions that exist within the field, and a sampling of traditional areas of investigation. Mann and Janelle then tackle the important role that attention plays across all aspects of sports endeavors. They note that irrespective of sport, ability level, or physical or cognitive demands, athletes must be able to focus attention on the right things at the right times. Successful athletes must be able to distinguish between internal and external distractions and relevant stimuli that are crucial for the proper execution of the skill or sports.

Coaches are central figures in the world of sports that are often revered or ascribed godlike status. Alternatively, they can be vilified and ridiculed when their team does not perform up to expectations. Vernacchia explores the psychosocial aspects of coaching and athletic leadership. He reviews important factors within the coach's world, the influence of the coach, the role of athletic leadership, the basic factors involved in effective coaching, and holistic coaching. Anyone who has had a coach can readily recognize the integral role coaches can play in the development of both athletic talent and personal excellence, while also understanding the negative consequences that arise as a result of poor or ineffective coaching.

Training leads to success. Therefore, train, train, train until you are exhausted, and then train again—not only today and tomorrow, but throughout the season, or even your career. The press for continuous training, even at very young ages, has become commonplace in sports. Raglin and Kenttä address the important question, "How long can these practices continue before records stop falling or athletes begin to break down?" They explore the notion of Overtraining Syndrome, which refers to the long-held observation that training regimens that improve performance for the majority of athletes may have deleterious effects for other individuals of equal skill and conditioning.

Identifying the personality profiles or characteristics that exemplify great athletes has been the Holy Grail for a great number of sports psychologists for many years. Given the widespread interest in this area, it would be reasonable to expect that sports psychology has a great deal to say on the subject. Webbe and his colleagues explore the core studies that have examined the relationship between personality variables and sports-related performance and behavior. Of particular interest are the personality factors that define risk of athletic injury as well as recovery from injury.

Russo and Marikle build on the foundation laid by Webbe et al. to further explore treatment, prevention, and understanding of the psychological ramifications of athletic injuries. The importance of this topic is underscored by the estimated 17 million people who are injured each year in sport- and exercise-related activities. Their chapter focuses on the psychological aspects of injuries sustained during sport and athletic activities, which is important to both the athletes who sustain the injuries and the sports medicine professionals who treat these athletes.

Bruce and Kym Burke then take us on a departure from the traditional research on sport psychology. Using their personal experiences from running a very successful gym, they identify the challenges, as well as some of the solutions, for becoming fit. They draw upon their experiences of working with a broad range of clients, ranging from the elderly to the elite athlete, inserting actual client experiences in order to reinforce their points. In a world filled with seemingly unending self-help volumes and a multibillion-dollar diet industry, they ask: Why have so many "failed" at exercise? What are the keys to a successful exercise experience? What does it mean to be healthy? What does it take to be fit?

Student-athletes are faced with tremendous amounts of pressure to compete, to be successful students, and to manage the various demands of their lives stoically and without complication. Vásquez Guerrero and his colleagues examine the unique challenges that student-athletes present to the sports medicine team. The clinically oriented sports psychologist must understand the crucible-like environment of pressures and relationships in which the athletes are expected to perform. They also must be cognizant of the developmental tasks and individual factors that impact a student-athlete's health, well-being, and performance. This chapter describes the university environment in which many student-athletes live and work, the developmental factors that mitigate or exacerbate psychopathology, and reviews approaches for assessing and treating student-athletes. The issues and intervention strategies that are discussed are applicable to athletes competing at all skill levels.

In a related although distinctly different topic area, Steinlight and Putukian examine what has been called the "Female Athlete Triad," which refers to the three interrelated components of amenorrhea, disordered eating, and osteoporosis. The importance of this chapter is underscored by the exponential increase in physical activity and sports participation among women. This chapter explores traditional definitions of the triad, the associated symptoms, effective interventions, and our current understanding of the spectrum that exists from health to disease.

Lastly, I explore and describe the emerging field of sport neuropsychology and the detection, treatment, and proper management of sports-related traumatic brain injury. At this time of this writing, there has been a virtual explosion in the popular media regarding the possible long-term consequences of sports-related brain injuries that may include relentless depression, dementia, and structural abnormalities in the brain. These concerns have led the U.S. Congress to conduct hearings into the National Football League's (NFL) management of concussions, and the NFL has made significant changes in its concussion management protocols. This chapter will describe the pathophysiology of concussion, the epidemiology of the injury, the signs and symptoms of concussion, current assessment methods, and the development of scientifically based return to play protocols.

Taken together, we hope that these chapters stimulate, excite, and leave you, the reader, asking for more. In doing so, we hope to energize your interest to explore this exciting area in greater detail, and to incorporate some of the principles and techniques in your own life to enhance your fitness, exercise, and sports participation.

Chapter 1

Sports Psychology: A Historical Overview

Ruben J. Echemendia

Sports psychology is a multidisciplinary research and applied science that traces its roots to philosophy, movement science, exercise science, psychology, and sociology, to name but a few. As a result of this amalgam of disciplines, sports psychology may be said to have "a long past but a short history." Indeed, Mahoney (1989) made an interesting observation when he described a paradox that exists with regard to sports psychology. He noted that although the conceptual roots of sports psychology can be traced to prehistoric antiquity, sports psychology has only recently become visible and popular. The goal of this chapter is to lay a historical foundation upon which the following chapters of this volume can be built. In doing so, this chapter will not present an exhaustive review of the historical literature, but rather a selected review where key areas are touched upon.

Broadly defined, sports psychology is the scientific study and application of psychological principles to athletic endeavors, including exercise and recreational/competitive sports. Williams and Straub (2006) further differentiate sports psychology by distinguishing among its component parts: "Applied sport psychology focuses on one facet of sports psychology, that of identifying and understanding psychological theories and interventions that can be applied to sports and exercise to enhance the performance of personal growth of athletes and physical activity participants" (p. 1). Psychological

interventions can take many forms and may be used to enhance positive experiences and promote positive mental health, or they can be
used to help ameliorate psychological disturbances such as anxiety
and depression. From the perspective of promoting positive performance characteristics, it has been argued that one important goal of
psychological interventions includes teaching athletes to consistently
create an ideal state of mind that will cause them to consistently chan-
nel their skills to achieve optimal performance. At a more basic level,
positive mental health can be enhanced and distressing psychological
symptoms minimized by the simple application of exercise, since it
has long been known that physical exercise has a positive effect on a
broad range of psychological and medical conditions. According to
Mahoney (1989), "In the case of Humans, the evidence is now quite
extensive: recreational play and athletics are integral to healthy
personality development, and they are very important elements of
societal and cultural development as well" (p. 110).

The roots of experimental sports psychology can be traced to the early
scientific investigations that focused on kinesthetics and reaction time.
It has been noted that "motor psychology" predated the emergence of
sports psychology by 50 years. Wiggins (1984) commented on the important and early contributions of Wilhelm Wundt in 1875, who, along with
his students, studied simple and complex reaction times. Although the
origins of moderate sports psychology have been traced to physical education and exercise science, some of the earliest and most influential scientific publications were conducted by psychologists who had
developed a special interest in sports and recreation.

Norman Triplett (1898), a student of Stanley Hall at Clark University, is widely regarded as having the first reported experiment in the
field of sports psychology. Interested in the area of social facilitation,
Triplett investigated bicycle racing and the winding of fishing reels
under conditions that were competitive and noncompetitive. He
found that paced races (more than one racer) were 25 percent faster
than those races in which there was only one racer. He then later confirmed these field observations in more controlled laboratory studies
where he used a reel winding paradigm. His body of research led to
early conclusions that individuals of all ages were positively stimu-
lated by the presence of others. He also noted that there were significant individual differences in how children react to competitive
circumstances, noting that 25 percent of his child sample had poor
performance in the competitive situations and occasionally "went to
pieces" at crucial times in the race (Wiggins, 1984). Triplett's work

provides an excellent early example of translational research whereby observations in the field are then reexamined under well-controlled laboratory conditions.

As we move ahead in time and across the Atlantic, there was great interest in the use of psychological principles and techniques in the development of peak performance. In 1921 a landmark book by Schulte in German focused on the psychological preparation of the elite athlete (*Increasing Performance and Exercises, Games, and Sport Activities*). Within the United States, Coleman Roberts Griffith, widely viewed as the founder of sports psychology, established the first laboratory for sports psychology research at the University of Illinois in 1925. Griffith focused on investigations related to athletes' reaction times and flexibility. He wrote two classic texts: *Psychology of Coaching* (1926) and *Psychology of Athletics* (1928). Griffith taught a course in sports psychology at the University of Illinois and helped to supervise graduate student research. Historical records indicate that he corresponded with legendary Notre Dame football coach Knute Rockne about psychological and motivational aspects of coaching and athletics. Griffith also served as team psychologist and researcher for the Chicago Cubs baseball team. Mahoney described an interesting story about Griffith: Griffith interviewed Harold E. ("Red") Grange, who scored four touchdowns in the first 12 minutes of the 1924 Illinois-Michigan football game. Two of his runs were returns of 95 and 67 yards. He was taken out of the game after his fourth touchdown, which Mahoney speculates may have been out of kindness to the Michigan team. Grange returned to the game in the fourth quarter, during which he ran for a fifth touchdown and passed 18 yards for a sixth. When Griffith interviewed Grange, he had no recall of any of his runs. He simply could not remember or describe any of his truly memorable plays. Grange's lack of memory for these events led Griffith to write about "automatic skill response." According to Mahoney, Griffith's observations regarding the automatic skills response laid the foundation for what has later been referred to as, "hot streak, groove, flow," or "sweet spot in time" (p. 103).

In the 1930s, Clarence Ragsdale at the University of Wisconsin became interested in motor learning. It has been observed that Ragsdale's textbook *The Psychology of Motor Learning* was the first textbook of its type in the United States. In his historical review, Wiggins (1984) indicates that other than the work of Ragsdale and investigations by Charles McCoy and his students at the University of Iowa, who were interested in the character and personality of athletes, and the work of Walter Miles from Stanford on reaction time among football players, very little empirical research surfaced in the U.S. literature relating to either motor learning or to sports psychology more generally prior to World War II.

Similarly, it appears that little research in this area occurred following Griffith's work and up until the 1960s, except for a book written by John Lawther in 1951 titled *Psychology of Coaching*. Lawther, at the University of Pennsylvania, provided coaches with particularly interesting observations on motivation, team cohesion, personality, feelings and emotions, and handling athletes. This book has been credited with starting the separation between studies in motor learning and sports psychology. During this time period there also appeared articles that examined the emotional reactions of football players versus wrestlers, and the study of stress during sport. After World War II, sports psychology began to flourish in the Soviet Union and Germany. In Japan in 1952, Mitsuo Matsui wrote *The Psychology of Physical Education* and helped establish sports psychology into the Japanese physical education curriculum (Wiggins, 1984).

Following World War II, the emphasis in the United States continued to be on motor learning. Motor learning laboratories were established at the University of California at Berkeley and at Indiana University, which awarded a PhD in physical education. In 1966, Ogilvie and Tutko published a volume entitled *Problem Athletes and How to Handle Them*, which came to the attention of many coaches because of their insights into athlete motivation. This text was an interesting collaboration between an American and a Czech that brought to Americans an understanding of applied clinical psychology as it was practiced in Eastern Europe with athletes and teams (Wiggins, 1984). Ogilvie has since been described as the founder of *applied* sports psychology in the United States.

Two important historical markers in the formal development of sports psychology occurred in the 1960s. The first congress of the International Society of Sports Psychology (ISSP) was held in Rome in 1965, attended by more than 400 participants who represented 27 countries (Williams & Straub, 2006). Under the leadership of Dr. Ferruccio Antonelli, an Italian, these meetings allowed scientists and practitioners to exchange views and research findings while understanding different cultural perspectives and their relation to sports psychology. In 1967, the Americans and Canadians joined forces to establish the North American Society for Psychology of Sports and Physical Activity (NASPSPA), which then hosted the second meeting of the ISSP in Washington, DC (1968). In 1969, Robert Wilberg at the University of Alberta founded the Canadian Society for Psychomotor Learning and Sports Psychology. Concurrently, sports psychology was developing in Europe, where the European Federation of Sport Psychology was created in 1969. Additional organizational development was noted in the 1970s with the emergence of sports psychology within the American College of Sports Medicine (ACSM) and the Sport Psychology Academy within the American Association for Health, Recreation and Physical Education (AAHPERD) in 1975. An initial goal of this group was to create links between research and practical application. In 1985, the Association for the Advancement of Applied Sport Psychology was formed by John Silva, and in 1987, the American Psychological Association officially recognized the Sports Psychology division, Division 47. Sports psychology organizations also proliferated throughout the world. For example, in the late 1960s, societies existed in Brazil, Czechoslovakia, the German Democratic Republic, France, Spain, England, the Scandinavian countries, and most of the countries of Eastern Europe, including Bulgaria, Romania, Hungary, and Poland (Wiggins, 1984).

The 1970s brought about significant interest and excitement in the area of sports psychology research. Sports psychology began to emerge as a science that relied on a programmatic and systemic body of research. Mahoney (1989) observed that sports psychology was being recognized in the mainstream media. After the 1976 Montréal Olympics, Mark Spitz stated in an interview that at the Olympic level of competition, physical skill differences were minimal relative to the importance of mental factors. Also adding fuel to the fire was a rumor that the Soviets employed more than 90 sports psychologists to help prepare their teams for the Montréal Olympics (Mahoney, 1989). During the 1984 Los Angeles Olympics, the American Broadcasting Company (ABC) showed a series of experts on the topic of sports psychology throughout its television coverage.

In 1978, the U.S. Olympic Committee (USOC) recruited expert advisors in four branches of sports science: biomechanics, exercise physiology, nutrition, and sports psychology. In 1983, the USOC established an official Sport Psychology Committee and a registry of qualified sport psychologists. The registry contained the names of individuals who were subjected to intensive review of their training and experience in the recognized three nonexclusive categories of sports psychologists: research, educational, and clinical (Mahoney, 1989). Research sports psychologists are primarily involved with testing theories and various conceptual models that explain or predict particular sport behaviors. Educational sports psychologists are typically involved in disseminating sports psychology knowledge. Clinical sports psychologists assist athletes who are experiencing psychological difficulties such as depression, anxiety, substance abuse, difficulties with interpersonal relationships, and situational life stress.

The 1980s were credited with the development of better documentation of the effectiveness of psychological interventions in performance enhancement. Similarly, increased attention was given to exercise and health psychology with a focus on issues such as exercise training, enhancing exercise programs, exercise addiction, injury response, rehabilitation, and the relationship between exercise and stress.

Paralleling the development of organized sports psychology was also the emergence of research journals that published the various investigational works of sports psychologists. At the start of the 1970s, there were two primary journals in sports psychology: The *International Journal of Sport Psychology*, which was first published in 1970, and the *Journal of Sports Psychology*, published in 1979. At about the same time, the *Canadian Journal of Applied Sport Sciences* emerged. In 1988, the title was changed to the *Journal of Sports and Exercise Psychology*. In 1987, the *Sport Psychologist* was published, and the *Journal of Applied Sport Psychology* appeared in 1989.

From 1990 until the present, there has been tremendous growth in the area of sports psychology, both in terms of its knowledge base and organizational structure, but also in further developing professional credentials in the field. In addition to traditional quantitative approaches that examined the effectiveness of interventions in performance enhancement, there has emerged a significant body of literature that relies on qualitative approaches to understanding sports psychology phenomena (Williams & Straub, 2006). Also of significance is the distinction between academic sports psychology and applied sports psychology. Academic sports psychology continues to be focused on the production of knowledge and research paradigms, whereas applied sports psychology seeks to apply the knowledge that has been developed in the clinical or real-life situation. This distinction led to the development of the Association for the Advancement of Applied Sports Psychology (AAASP), and the *Journal of Applied Sport Psychology* became the official publication of the AAASP with its inaugural publication in March 1989 (Cox, Qiu, & Liu, 1993).

Any overview of the historical foundations of sports psychology would not be complete without recognizing the schism that occurred in the field between "psychology" and "exercise science" and between the scientists and the applied practitioners. These divides are not new to psychology, or science more generally. There has always been friction between "basic" scientists and the applied fields. This has been notable within psychology, most obviously in the areas of clinical psychology and industrial-organizational psychology. Even within disciplines, these divides are often apparent. For example, clinical neuropsychology continues to struggle with the relationships among its basic scientists and academics on one hand, and the more applied clinical practitioners on the other. Within APA, there was a schism between the "academics and scientists" and the practitioners, in part leading to the creation of the American Psychological Society.

Wiggins (1984) described the tension that has existed between those with backgrounds in physical education with little experience in psychology, and those with certification in clinical psychology who have entered the field with little or no background in sports psychology research. "Psychologists on the other hand, point out that the physical educators working in the field are not really psychologists at all. Thus, these psychologists say, physical educators may be able to talk *about* athletes and psychology, but they should not talk *to* athletes about their own psyches!" (p. 23). Feltz and Kontos have argued that the distinction between sports psychology as a subdiscipline of psychology or a subdiscipline of exercise science is not trivial. Their view is that the choice of the parent discipline has important implications for the direction of the field. They provide the following examples: As a subdiscipline of psychology, sports psychology will likely focus on understanding psychological theories and applying psychological principles. As a subdiscipline of sport and exercise science, sports psychology's focus would be on "trying to describe, explain, and predict behavior in sports contexts" (p. 4).

In response to the many professional and ethical issues in the field, AAASP developed a model curriculum in 1991 for certification by AAASP for individuals who provide performance enhancement services. The criteria include a doctoral degree that encompasses knowledge from the disciplines of psychology and kinesiology, the equivalent of 3 courses in sports psychology, training in professional ethics and standards, and supervised practica with a qualified individual. In 1994, the supervision criteria was made more stringent, requiring 400 hours; and in 2002, a process for certifying individuals with a master's degree was set forth. Certification and licensing of clinically oriented sports psychologists is governed by the individual state licensing boards and the APA's Ethical Guidelines for psychologists. Commenting on the distinction between applied sports psychology and research sports psychology Cox, Qiu, and Liu (1993) stated, "Academic and applied sport psychologists must never lose sight of the fact that working together will be more effective than working separately" (p. 4). Indeed, it is likely that neither would exist in today's funding climate without the other and that both together could fashion a more complete discipline than either alone.

Thus far we have focused on important historical developments within sports psychology. In the pages that follow, we will shift our attention toward highlighting key areas of investigation within sports psychology. As with the previous section of this chapter, what follows is by no means an exhaustive review of the literature in sports psychology, but rather an attempt to acquaint the reader with some important historical areas of investigation. The organization of domains that follows is based on Mahoney's (1989) classification of research areas.

PERSONALITY

Central to the study of modern sports psychology has been the goal of understanding and describing the psychological profile or psychological makeup of elite athletes. Underlying this focus is the belief that great athletes possessed personality traits or psychological profiles that could be distinguished from those who are less talented. Similarly, there was the belief that great leaders could be reliably distinguished from their less successful peers. Several instruments were used in an attempt to identify a general athletic personality—for example, the Minnesota Multiphasic Personality Inventory (MMPI), the California Psychological Inventory (CPI), the Maudsley Personality Inventory (MPI), and the Cattell 16 PF IPAT (Mahoney, 1989). The use of these instruments, which were largely designed to measure patterns of psychopathology, created a camp that was known as the sport "personologists." This research paradigm was criticized by others who viewed it as research devoid of theory and those who sought to emphasize psychological skills rather than enduring traits. Indeed, Morgan suggested, "if all research design flaws were removed from sport personality research studies, a significant but slight relationship could be observed between athletic performance and personality testing" (Cox, Qui, & Liu, 1993). More recently, psychologists have begun to adopt an interactionistic perspective that recognizes the relationships among enduring personality traits and psychological skills that are modifiable through various intervention techniques. Morgan is credited with having identified patterns of positive mental health or positive indicators of personality that were associated with successful athletes. He identified the "iceberg profile" using the Profile of Mood States (POMS), which revealed that elite athletes scored relatively low on tension, depression, anger, fatigue, and confusion while scoring higher on vigor when compared to the general population. Morgan did warn, however, against the use of the POMS in the selection of athletes. A landmark study by Schurr, Ashley, and Joy (1977) investigated 1,596 college students (athletes and nonathletes) who completed the Cattell 16 PF questionnaire. They found significant relationships between athletes and nonathletes and between athletes of individual sports and those involved in team sports.

PSYCHOLOGICAL SKILLS

Mahoney, Gabriel, and Perkins (1987) found that elite athletes reported being more highly motivated to do well and more reliant on internally referenced and kinesthetic (whole body and internal imagery) mental preparations than their less successful peers. The elite group also reported fewer problems with performance anxiety, greater success and concentration during competition, and higher levels of self-confidence.

AROUSAL/ANXIETY

The famous Yerkes-Dodson inverted-U hypotheses states that very low and very high levels of arousal are associated with poor performance, while moderate levels of arousal are associated with better performance. This model has received substantial support in the literature and has been associated with Eastbrooks's cue utilization theory, which posits that attention narrows as arousal increases. Narrowing of attention allows the athlete to focus on relevant cues while ignoring or not being distracted by irrelevant cues.

The performance anxiety and stress associated with competition and public performance have been at the forefront of athletes' concerns and a common focus of sport psychologists. Cox, Qui, and Lui's (1993) review of the literature identifies two important general findings regarding precompetitive anxiety. They note that experienced athletes differ from less experienced athletes, with experienced athletes tending to reach their peak levels of anxiety at a different time than less experienced athletes. Second, they note that precompetitive anxiety takes the form of an inverted V, where anxiety begins to build as the competition nears and continues to build until just prior to the start of the athletic event. As the event gets near a sudden drop in the anxiety occurs immediately prior to the start of the event. This pattern of precompetitive anxiety has been noted to be higher for individual sport athletes and team athletes. It has also been noted that differences in the type of anxiety, whether somatic or cognitive anxiety, differentially affect athletic performance. Research has also underscored that there are significant individual differences and preferences with respect to pre-performance anxiety and that, "it is likely that the absolute level of anxiety may be less important than the personal meaning of that anxiety, as well as what the athlete does in relationship to it" (Mahoney, 1989). Research also suggests that peak performers are less likely to experience their anxiety as an "enemy," and they appear to be less susceptible to "anxiety-induced anxiety," which Mahoney describes as panicking over how anxious they feel. Research focused on interventions aimed at reducing anxiety or better managing anxiety has revealed several efficacious techniques including relaxation strategies, autogenic training, hypnosis, mental imagery, and cognitive behavioral interventions.

CONCENTRATION SKILLS

Peak performers appear to have developed exceptional concentration abilities that vary according to sport. The phenomenon of "flow" has been studied extensively. The characteristics of the flow experience include: "(1) It is experienced as an altered state of consciousness in which an unusual body-brain integration is achieved. (2) There is often a sense of timelessness. (3) Even during strenuous exercise, there is a sense of effortlessness sometimes described as being on automatic pilot. (4) Becoming aware of and/or trying to control the flow (e.g., trying to extend it) often results in its disappearance. (5) Flow is something that can be allowed to happen, but even the most successful athletes report an inability to produce it at will" (Mahoney, 1989, p. 116).

Studies have indicated that attentional processes or concentration skills may serve a crucial role in the flow phenomena. Data obtained from Elite riflery experts revealed that these experts spontaneously developed the ability to detect their own heartbeat and that, at peak levels of performance, they were pulling the trigger just before ventricular contractions (Mahoney, 1989). Marathon runners displayed similar high levels of focused attention. It has been reported that these athletes often cognitively dissociate from sensory input during training and competition, which allows them to dissociate pain stimuli and get past the "wall." Mahoney provides interesting examples such as the runner who reported that he performed a review of his life during each race, beginning with the first grade and then reviewing his memories of each and every year thereafter. Another runner wrote letters to family and friends in his head, while a third runner listened to Beethoven in his head. Individual strategies varied in content, but they all served to foster dissociation.

CONFIDENCE

According to Bandura, the most important predictor for enhanced self-confidence is successful performance. Following this model, the role of teachers and coaches is to engage in "participatory modeling," which provides the athlete with success experiences rather than failure. Fairly consistent evidence suggests that more successful athletes tend to be more highly confident. It appears the confidence is a highly personalized experience, with both general and specific correlates. It is important to keep in mind however that elite competitors rarely report absolute levels of confidence with an absence of self doubts. Elite athletes often report experiencing hesitation and doubts as they approach challenges. The distinction may be that self-confident elite athletes have greater willingness or even a strong desire to risk competition. Elite athletes may also have a perspective on competition that helps them to distinguish the importance of competitive outcomes and their worth as a person. In other words, their success or failure on the athlete field may be less tied to their value as a person. In this sense, the focus is more on the process of the competition or the desire to achieve optimal form than on the outcome of the competition per se. According to Mahoney (1989), individuals who "remain faithful to themselves—positive and affirming in their self regard irrespective of any specific successes and failures—may ironically be more likely to render more exceptional performances."

MOTIVATION

Skill, arousal, and training lay the groundwork for successful athletic performance, but little can be accomplished without appropriate goals and purpose. Athletes' self-reports generally reflect that reasonable and personally meaningful goals enhance training, whereas goals that are seen as arbitrary or unreasonable are deleterious to peak performance. The study of motivation has incorporated mediating variables such as perceived ability, self-efficacy, and achievement orientation. Overall, the motivation to participate in sports likely changes along with changes in life circumstances, and the meaning of success may change the very process of becoming successful. Mahoney has observed that contrary to the image often portrayed by the media, athletes who drive themselves single-mindedly towards improvement may actually perform less well than those whose quest for improvement exists within a more balanced perspective of life's priorities. Also of significance is that athletes and coaches alike have become aware that motivational slumps may be a result of overtraining and athletes pushing themselves too hard.

MENTAL PREPARATIONS

The mental preparations performed by athletes in anticipation of actual competition may be divided into two nonexclusive areas of study: Those having to do with last-minute preparations and those focusing on mental rehearsal, mental practice, and imagery (Mahoney, 1989). Last-minute preparations vary considerably as a function of individual differences in both the content and the effectiveness of the strategies. For some athletes, pre-competition rituals may alter the extent of their physiological arousal, confidence, or concentration. Other athletes may use the pre-competition rituals to help them feel centered and more highly focused on their performance.

Mental practice or mental rehearsal has been widely studied in sport psychology. As is true for many areas of psychology, the findings have at times been contradictory and confusing. Taken together, these studies suggest that on average, mentally rehearsing a performance can be beneficial, particularly if the athlete has prior knowledge and experience with the task and can perform it at moderate skill levels. It appears that mental practice combined with physical practice may better than either alone. Exceptional athletes appear to engage in a whole-body form of mental practice, "rehearsing not only what they might see during a performance but also the feeling of their movements, as well as the sounds and smells of the competition" (Mahoney, 1989, p. 119).

TEAM COHESION

A significant amount of research has focused on the issue of team cohesion. There is little question that a significant positive relationship exists between successful athletic performance and team cohesion. The research in this area seems to suggest that cooperation within a team is superior to competition within a team in terms of both cooperation and productivity. Cox, Qui, and Lui (1993) observed that team members who cooperate with each other in order to attain team goals are much more likely to be successful than those team members who seek individual goals at the expense of team goals and objectives. A relationship also exists between the nature of the task and levels of cooperation and competition. In situations where significant team-mate interaction is required, the more important cooperation becomes for successful outcome.

In closing, this chapter has attempted to provide the reader with an overview of the field of sports psychology by examining its historical roots, delineating key aspects of the development of discipline, briefly pointing out areas of tension, and then selectively highlighting some key areas of research. Sports psychology is clearly a dynamic and multidisciplinary area that is relatively young in its developmental trajectory. As sports and exercise continue to play an increasingly important role in our lives, across all ages and ability levels, sports psychology will continue to enjoy growth and visibility as long as there is respect and cooperation among the many different perspectives and traditions that encompass the sports psychology team.

REFERENCES AND RECOMMENDED READING

Cox, R. H., Qiu, Y. & Liu, Z. (1993). Overview of sport psychology. In R. N. Singer, M. Murphey, & L. K. Tennant (Eds.), *Handbook of research on sport psychology* (pp. 3–31). New York: Macmillan Publishing.

Mahoney, M. J. (1989). Sport psychology. In I. S. Cohen (Ed.), *The G. Stanley Hall lecture series*, vol. 9 (pp. 97–134). Washington, DC: American Psychological Association.

Wiggins, D. K. (1984). The history of sport psychology. In J. M. Silva & R. S. Weinberg (Eds.), *Psychological foundations of sport* (pp. 8–27). Champaign, IL: Human Kinetics.

Williams, J. M. & Straub, W. F. (2006). Sport psychology: past, present and future. In J. M. Williams (Ed.), *Applied sport psychology: Personal growth to peak performance* (pp. 1–14). New York: McGraw Hill.

Chapter 2

Optimizing Attentional Allocation and Sport Performance Using the Five-step Strategy

Derek T. Y. Mann and Christopher M. Janelle

Elite athletic performance requires consistent, extensive, and systematic training over long periods of time during which several domains of expertise are developed. Such domains include physical, technical, cognitive, and emotional skills. While the determination of how such skills are developed remains a vibrant area for sports psychology research, it is clear that expert athletes must master sport-specific skills that fall in each of these domains to realize high-level performance in any sport. Such demands are extensive and widely differentiated among sports. While certain sports may require heavy reliance on muscular endurance, others may require supreme physical strength. Coordinated efforts among teammates will influence competition outcome in team sports, while an individual's ability to maintain high levels of training in solitude will dictate success in many individual sport settings.

From a psychological standpoint, athletes must pay attention to the right things at the right time to be successful. Regardless of the type of sport, the level at which the sport is played, or the physical and cognitive demands of the task, the need to direct attention to the most critical (information-rich) areas in the environment, and the ability to ignore

internal and external distractions while maintaining appropriate allocation of attention is undeniable.

Indeed, it is reasonable to assert that attention is *the most critical proximal* predictor of performance outcome, spawning the question: What
are the right things to pay attention to, and when is the right time to
pay attention? Broadly, the right things refer to the most important
information-gathering aspects of the internal and external environment. Timing is everything, however. Cues that are relevant one
moment may be completely irrelevant the next. In the former sense,
they should be attended, while they should be ignored in the latter.
Clearly then, to develop expertise in sports, one must either implicitly
or explicitly acquire knowledge concerning what are the most important cues present in the specific sport context, and when to attend to
them. The purpose of this chapter is to help athletes to become aware
of the critical cues in their sports, to gain an appreciation and awareness
of the sources of distraction that can detract from quality practice and
competition, and to present a context within which the mental game
can be couched to increase the likelihood of being able to pay attention
to the right things at the right time.

A CONTEXTUAL MODEL FOR THE ROLE
AND IMPORTANCE OF ATTENTION

Coaches, athletes, and sports psychologists (both researchers and
practitioners) might argue with the assertion that attentional focus is
the paramount psychological skill that must be mastered for elite performance. What about motivation? Confidence? Emotion regulation?
Mental toughness? These are each critical in their own right, along
with all of the perceptual, emotional, and strategic aspects of their
performance. However, each of these mental skills, though critical,
are comparatively *distal* predictors of performance (Figure 2.1).

In other words, it is what each of these psychological skills influence
that determine performance, and *what they influence is attention*. Not sur-
prisingly, therefore, attention has routinely been shown to differentiate
experts and nonexperts across a range of sports and other achievement
domains.

Theorists differ widely in their perspectives of what attention is and
what aspects of attention are critical. While perspectives differ, it is
generally agreed that attention is *limited*; there is only so much attention
that can be allocated at any given moment. Attention to something (or
several things) inherently means that those attentional resources cannot

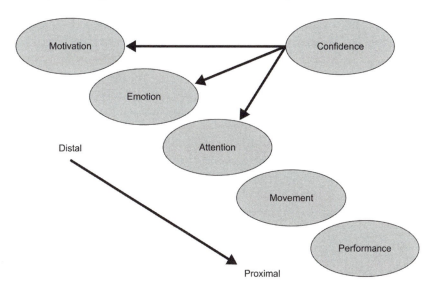

Figure 2.1.   A contextual model of distal to proximal temporal influences on sport performance.

be directed elsewhere. Well-learned skills become highly automated, requiring less attentional resources to do the same work that was done prior with more resources. Resources, indeed the neurons themselves, become highly specialized, and function becomes increasingly localized in the brain, an adaptive process that inherently permits the performer to use available resources for performance of other tasks. For example, as a basketball player automizes the ability to dribble the basketball without "thinking about it," the player's attentional reserves increase for allocation to the external environment, permitting her or him to survey the defense, ascertain how a play might develop, and be able to narrow in on the openings that are offered by the defense to pass the ball, shoot it, or drive for the basket. More specifically, strategic options become the focus of attention rather than directing attention toward regulation of movements needed to dribble the basketball.

Such an adaptive process of attention as individuals traverse from relative novice to expert in sport has been studied for many years now, yielding a rich database from which to draw inferences as to what sports psychologists should be striving for to manifest optimal attentional focus among athletes across numerous sports. This database has been assimilated using a variety of methods and measures but has largely occurred in the context of the expert-novice protocol. Such a protocol involves comparison of experts in a sport to those who are either novice or near expert and then ascertaining how they differ on a particular response measure. Popular assessments of attention using the expert-novice paradigm include such measures as eye tracking, brain wave recording, behavioral, and self-report indices. While aspects of attention that are specific to different sports vary, the extant research to date clearly indicates that:

1. Expert athletes attend to the most important information-rich areas of a visual display, thereby inhibiting attention to unimportant or distracting areas.

2. Expert brains adapt to the task demands that are specific to the sports they play. Expert marksmen, for example, demonstrate favorable activation of different hemispheres of the brain, and specific locations in the brain, that in turn highlight the need for maximal visuospatial processing and minimal interference from verbal and analytical processes.

3. Experts maintain visual focus for longer periods of time on relevant cues, with final fixations to targets being significantly longer than their nonexpert counterparts.

4. Expert emotional states appear to lead to more favorable attentional changes as compared to nonexperts.

5. Experts are less distractible by internal factors, such as negative thoughts, worries, and concerns.

6. Experts are more attentionally flexible, permitting them to disengage irrelevant cues and engage relevant ones in time to make the appropriated decisions.

7. Experts are faster at recognizing task-specific patterns and anticipating opponents actions due to greater vigilance and lesser distractibility.

8. Experts are more effective, efficient, and often perform with less effortful than their less skilled counterparts.

Relying on the considerable database that describes the attentional conditions that yield the expert advantage, sports psychologists now have greater knowledge than ever concerning what attentional conditions are optimal for many sports and classes of sport skills. Relying on this knowledge, the sports psychologist aims to help novice athletes acquire attentional states that reflect those of their higher-skilled counterparts. For example, each sport demands attention, but the demands of each sport require specific and unique attention skills so the athlete can attend to the most task-relevant features (e.g., preparatory activities or performance environment) at the most appropriate time.

An athlete's ability to shift attention and focus on task-relevant cues is fundamental to success. Practically speaking, attention in sport can be conceptualized as the interaction between the width and direction of one's attention/focus. Width of attention is best understood as broad or narrow, while direction refers to internal or external. For example, a pitcher in baseball will determine what pitch to throw in a given context (i.e., broad-internal) but should switch to a narrow-external focus of attention (catcher's mitt) to free performance from conscious processing. So, how does a sports psychologist help an aspiring athlete to assume the attentional states that are most ideal for the sports they play? Let's examine a few different sports and discuss the attentional requirements for each prior to offering answers to that question:

Golf requires extreme levels of highly focused concentration, but for rather short periods of time. In a 4-hour round of golf, an individual will typically spend about 5 minutes or so actually hitting the golf ball. Herein lies the difficulty for golfers—an inordinate amount of time that the mind is free to wander (and arguably should) coupled with an extraordinary amount of time available to worry about a poor shot or bask in a good one. All shots in golf are self-paced, but other environmental factors can compromise shot selection and predictability from time to time.

Tennis is another example of a sport that is marked with extensive periods of inaction—time to think, and potentially to think of irrelevant things. The typical point does not last very long, with plenty of time between points for the mind to wander, refocus, and continue. Also, time exists between every other game that can be used adaptively to mentally prepare for the next two games, or not. Attentional demands of tennis vary from self-paced, highly predictable acts, such as serving the ball, to extremely reactive, highly unpredictable demands, as exemplified by serves that can travel upwards of 150 mph.

Auto racing: The attentional demands of a sport like auto racing are quite different from those required for and exhibited in golf or tennis. Highly focused attention is required for the duration of the race, with very few breaks for lapses of attention, which

occur only during a pit stop or a yellow flag; even then, attention must be allocated to making adjustments to the race car,
strategy, etc. Indeed, there is arguably no sport that requires a
greater amount of highly focused attention over such an
extended period of time.

Interactive team sports: While auto racing requires teamwork for
success, the attentional demands of other sports such as baseball, hockey, basketball, and football, for example, require a vast
array of attentional skills that range from snippets of highly
focused, short-term attentional allocation to opportunities for
attentional lapses, to extreme and enduring attentional bouts.

Running and other endurance sports: The casual observer may not be
aware of the attentional demands faced by runners and other
endurance athletes, and they are certainly different among
endurance sports. It is quite clear that the favored strategy for
elite athletes is one in which associative attentional strategies
are favored (and arguably mandated) over dissociative ones.

In sum, numerous aspects of attention have been studied over the
years, permitting the development of a rich database that has documented the attentional demands of specific sports and the individuals
who excel in them. Such attentional requirements must be met for
successful performance, regardless of the very clear differences in
attentional requirements among sports. As sports psychologists, one
of our primary objectives is to aid in the ability to develop an ideal
approach to yield the most adaptive attentional strategies that will give
the athlete the best opportunity to be successful. However, it is important to realize that implementation of an attention-focusing control
strategy cannot occur in the absence of consideration of other aspects
of the mental approach that are critical for performance. Indeed, optimizing motivational orientations, emotional states, and mental practice
will aid in the development of an ideal attentional strategy. Context
matters and is the focus of our next segment.

A FRAMEWORK FOR TRAINING AND IMPLEMENTING
ATTENTIONAL SKILLS

Preperformance routines have been associated with "closed-tasks"
and self-paced activities for which specific behaviors (i.e., number of
ball bounces or golf club "waggles") and thoughts (imagery of task,

outcome, positive mood words, etc.) performed immediately prior to performance are believed to regulate thoughts and emotions, increase preparedness, and enhance performance. The preparatory routine is often referred to as a "psyching-up" strategy, is used by athletes to alter their physiological arousal level and direct their attention to the ensuing task. Unfortunately, most athletes engage in an unsystematic conglomeration of thoughts, physical activities, and/or rituals with the hope of bettering their performance.

The best preparatory routines are those in which every aspect of the routine has a purpose. The benefits of systematic preparatory routines have been demonstrated across a variety of sports, most notably golf putting, basketball free-throw shooting, running speed, power lifting, gymnastics, marksmanship, archery, and swimming, among others. Research has supported the notion that to be effective, preparatory routines should consist of a systematic sequencing of task-relevant thoughts and actions that are executed immediately prior to performance. An effective routine will in turn facilitate the readiness of the athlete by maximizing arousal, confidence, and attentional focus in the moments leading up to performance.

THE FIVE-STEP STRATEGY

Singer's five-step strategy is one example of a context in which to embed several psychological skills that will lead to creation of an optimal preparatory routine. Preparatory routines can be directed toward an extended period of preparation, such as an entire day of competition, or can be very short-lived and specific, such as the preshot routine that a golfer or basketball player performs prior to a putt or free throw, respectively. As alluded to, every aspect of the routine has meaning, and arguably, the meaning of the routine is to permit execution of the desired movement the right way at the right time. If we return to the notion that attentional focus is the paramount proximal psychological skill, we must consider the effect of the distal factors of performance such as motivation, confidence, and emotion regulation on performance.

The five-step strategy is a preparatory routine that encompasses the systematic execution of task-relevant thoughts and behaviors designed to elicit the most effective thoughts and emotions requisite for optimal performance. Inclusive are the many psychological components underlying attention allocation, including, motivation, confidence, and emotion regulation.

The five steps include:

1. *Readying.* Establishing a routine that involves optimal positioning of the body, confidence, expectations, and emotions.
2. *Imaging.* The creation of a mental image and the associated feelings of performing at one's best.
3. *Focusing Attention.* Directing thoughts to a relevant external cue or thought.
4. *Executing.* Performing the task with a quiet mind, free from distraction.
5. *Evaluating.* Assessing the quality of task execution, outcome, and the quality of the pre-performance strategy.

Given that the depth, breadth, and quality of attention have been shown to directly affect the quality of performance and that the distal predictors of performance can have a direct impact on attention, each of these components are addressed under the guise of the five-step strategy.

Readying

The interaction between perception and emotion has been supported across a variety of sporting tasks (e.g., martial arts, driving, billiards, biathlon shooting), suggesting that as anxiety increases, a corresponding reduction in the accuracy and efficiency of information processing and task performance is likely. It is a commonly held belief that anxiety leads to attentional narrowing, such that the breadth of attention is reduced and distractibility is increased, often resulting in delayed or impaired decision making and movement execution. However, under periods of heightened anxiety, a mobilization of additional attentional resources is likely to occur in an effort to offset the effects of anxiety to sustain a desired level of decision-making accuracy, often at the expense of decision-making speed. In some cases, performance is merely less efficient, while at other times, performance becomes impaired due to delayed processing speed.

When the outcome of an ensuing event is uncertain, athletes typically experience elevated levels of stress, arousal, and anxiety. Consequently, the highly complex, competitive, and unpredictable nature of sport often prompts heightened arousal and anxiety. According to Attentional Control Theory and its predecessor, Processing Efficiency Theory, the interaction of individual state and trait levels of anxiety coupled with environmental constraints (e.g., performance pressure and/or uncertainty) directly impact attentional capacity. Specifically, the capacity and resilience of the short-term working memory (i.e., the temporary storage of information essential for linking perception and action) is strongly dependent on attention and inherently limits human information processing. Short-term working memory is thus susceptible to the adverse effects of increased state anxiety, which can compromise performance. Cognitive anxiety, which is characterized by worry and an inability to concentrate, can thereby redirect attention toward a preoccupation with thoughts of evaluation and outcome expectations, and away from task relevant cues. As anxiety increases, however, performance decrements may be avoided via the recruitment and allocation of additional cognitive resources. While requiring increased effort, performance level will be sustained. Beyond a certain threshold, the allocation of additional resources can no longer counteract the negative affects of performance, and performance declines (Figure 2.2).

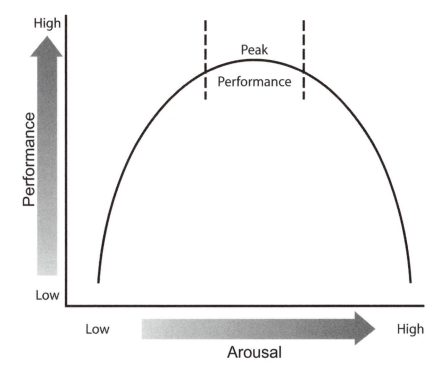

Figure 2.2.   Arousal performance relationship reflecting the importance of matching contextual arousal with task demands for maximizing sport performance.

To manage the potential detrimental effects of anxiety on performance, the readying stage places emphasis on maintaining and optimizing the emotional state, level of confidence, and performance expectations of the athlete, all of which have resounding effects on managing anxiety while maximizing performance. The temporal window prior to performance execution can prove instrumental to performance success. During the readying stage, the athlete should attend to and regulate the following three components: confidence, emotions, and expectations.

Emotions

Given the level of performance uncertainty that accompanies highly competitive and challenging tasks, corresponding increases in stress, arousal, and anxiety are expected. The interaction of individual state and trait levels of anxiety coupled with performance pressure directly impact the functional capacity of attention, rendering performance less efficient and potentially less effective. Cognitive anxiety, which is characterized by worry and an inability to concentrate, diverts thoughts and cognitions away from task-relevant cues and preoccupies cognitions with outcome expectations and evaluation. Elevated levels of cognitive anxiety reduce the capacity of working memory necessary to sustain task-relevant processing and may in turn result in the athlete directing attention inward, attending to the mechanics of the skill and away from critical performance cues. In other words, the more an athlete worries, the more he or she uses attentional resources, which likely decreases performance.

Contrary to intuitive expectations, not all negative emotions are detrimental to performance. Every athlete is unique in his or her desired direction and intensity of emotion experienced prior to and during a competition. For example, some athletes may prefer to feel anxious and energetic, while others may prefer to feel quiet and carefree, but in both cases the athletes are in their optimal performance state. As a result, the readying stage is intended to provide an opportunity for the athlete to regulate and evoke the most conducive emotional state to maximize performance. Individual athletes will benefit from identifying their own individual mental set that provides the best psychological and physiological (physical) conditions conducive to total task involvement and the recruitment of maximum resources for optimal performance. This state will vary from one athlete to another. For one athlete, the feelings of anxiety prior to a big point may signal the importance of the point, fully engaging the athlete. On the other hand, the same level of anxiety may overwhelm another athlete, leading to distraction and less-than-ideal performance. Identification of the most appropriate approach proceeds over time through systematic practice and routine introspection.

Key to effective implementation of the five-step strategy is that athletes learn how to recognize the different emotions that he or she may experience prior to and during competition, and how these emotions affect performance. Without awareness of the effect of performance fluctuations due to emotional states, it is virtually impossible to determine how to regulate current emotions to yield desired results. The athlete should look to identify the optimal combination of emotions and their respective intensity levels to elicit optimal performance. Identifying the corresponding signs of increased arousal and anxiety and how personal and situational factors affect both emotion and attention are critical. Lastly, the athlete should learn how to best cope with different situations while being skilled at eliciting the optimal emotions for maximum performance.

Given that the readying stage provides an opportunity for the athlete to evoke the necessary emotions, both direction (positive or negative) and intensity for maximum performance, during this stage the athlete may benefit from incorporating one or more of the following techniques to assist in achieving the ideal performance state.

1. *Progressive Muscle Relaxation (PMR)*: Although PMR is not a direct intervention for redirecting attention to task-relevant cues, the reduction in tension and anxiety may free the mind and body by becoming less distracting. In turn more resources are may be available to process task-relevant cues. PMR involves a sequential contracting a relaxing of the muscles of the body to relieve the muscle of excess tension. Away from competition, the athlete may choose to engage every muscle, working from the tips of one's toes to the top of one's head to maximize relaxation, rest, and recovery. Immediately prior to a competition or even during a competition, PMR can be equally effective at reducing tension. The maximal contraction of the large muscles of the body will help reduce tension and anxiety. This behavior can impact energy management and ultimately attention.

2. *Breath Control*: Similar to PMR, breath control is another relaxation technique that can have an indirect effect on attention by reducing anxiety and muscle tension. When muscle tension and anxiety

increase, breathing becomes truncated, increasing core tension while contributing to the internal distractibility of anxiety and muscle tension. However, conscious effort to engage in deep, rhythmical breathing allows the muscles of the core to elongate, promoting relaxation. As a result, the physical release of tension can translate into a quiet mind; a mental state more conducive to performance excellence.

3. *Self-talk/Mood Words*: Although self-talk has the potential to be an internal distracter (i.e., self-deprecating dialogue), when used effectively, self-talk can play an instrumental role in evoking an optimal mood state while redirecting attention toward task-relevant environmental cues. Most athletes engage in some form of internal dialogue. Unfortunately, this dialogue is often self-deprecating or entails the conscious processing of a well-learned skill. In either event, such dialogue is counterproductive. Self-talk can take on many forms, including instructional, motivational, mood enhancing, and confidence building. However, research suggests that self-talk should be task-specific. For example, for skill-based tasks, instructional self-talk has been shown to be most beneficial. Motivational self-talk is most effective for strength-based tasks. In either case, self-talk can be an effective strategy for managing emotions while redirecting attention to critical cues.

4. *Thought Stoppage*: When used in conjunction with self-talk, thought stoppage is a tremendously effective strategy for inter-vening with negative thoughts before they impact performance. Simply, thought stoppage requires the athlete to recognize when negative dialogue occurs, embrace the dialogue momentarily; just long enough to interrupt the thought with a cue word (i.e., stop) or behavior (i.e., tap of your racquet). Once the negative thought has been disrupted, the use of positive self-talk will help redirect attention back to the task at hand and away from the del-eterious effects of self-deprecating dialogue.

Imaging

Perhaps the most diverse mental skill for coaches and athletes is that of mental imagery. Imagery as part of preparatory routine has been noted to influence arousal regulation, attentional focus, confidence, and overall quality of performance. The popularity of imagery among elite athletes as a component of training and preperformance routines is profound. Jack Nicklaus, arguably one of the greatest golfers of all time, frequently was quoted:

> I never hit a shot, not even in practice, without having a very sharp, in-focus picture of it in my head. First I see the ball where I want it to finish, nice and white and sitting up high on the bright green grass. Then the scene quickly changes, and I see the ball going there: its path, trajectory, and shape, even its behavior on landing. Then there is a sort of fade-out, and the next scene shows me making the kind of swing that will turn the previous images into reality.

Surveys of Olympic gymnasts revealed that 92 percent of the participants used imagery to rehearse sport-specific skills, regulate emotions, set goals, and enhance concentration. In a survey of Canadian Olympic athletes, it was reported that 99 percent of those assessed indicated using imagery regularly in training and as a preparation strategy for competition. Surveys and testimonials advocate the use of imagery. The addition of imagery to any athlete's repertoire may prove invaluable.

Mental imagery refers to the process of creating or recreating an experience in one's mind and engaging the senses as if the activity was physically experienced. Sport scientists have identified a number of possible explanations as to why this mental re-creation proves useful, providing a framework for which imagery may be developed and incorporated into the five-step strategy to enhance attention and performance.

One explanation is derived from the work of psychologists who study the complex workings of the human body. These sports psycho-physiologists have developed the functional equivalence model, which suggests that the mind sends signals to the body that resemble those experienced while physically performing a task. In this case, although the body is relatively stationary, the muscles fire in the same sequential patterning, but free from physical exertion. Research with downhill skiers demonstrated that recorded muscle activity in-task coincided with specific turns and jumps while the athlete imaged skiing the course.

Others believe that imagery benefits performance symbolically. Through imagery, skills are coded in the mind and are recalled systematically during future performances. Simply put, imaging a task enhances the systematic process for which the motor programs can be recalled, leading to automaticity. In either case, imagery is linked to performance enhancement through priming. Attention is directed to the task, including a response-orientation that effectively primes the athlete both mentally and physically for the ensuing performance. This "priming" of the neuromuscular pathways helps to increase the probability of movement accuracy by reinforcing the coordination of the action, and further reduces the attentional demands placed on the athlete, freeing additional resources to account for other environmental demands.

From a cognitive behavioral perspective, the effectiveness of imagery can be accounted for via information processing models that include how information is acquired, processed, stored, and retrieved. It has been suggested that imagery has utility emitted through information gathered from the environment that will in turn elicit particular emotional responses that can be modified to enhance future performance. For example, a golfer may get overly anxious prior to hitting their first tee shot, often resulting in a less-than-ideal outcome. According to this theory, imagery provides an opportunity to re-create this environment while regulating the emotions experienced and optimizing the expected outcome. As a result, attention is allocated to external cues such as the target and away from a conscious processing of instructional cues in the moments prior to execution. Redirecting attention away from the internal cues tied to feeling anxious and toward the effects of the movements (i.e., ball flight, hitting the target, etc.) permits greater automatic processing.

The main difference between imagery and physically performing the task itself is the intensity of the muscular patterning, and that the emotional response during a task can be re-created and dealt with effectively or modified altogether. Although there are different theoretical explanations for how imagery works, the notion that preperformance imagery is intended to facilitate the preparatory state of the athlete is best exemplified by combining the elements of each theory, resulting in an inclusive and diversified program.

There is a necessary and natural progression of steps required to establish an efficient and effective imagery program. These instructions can be used as a checklist and were developed to enhance the imagery experience:

1. *Attention to the Task*: Decide on the critical components of your performance for which you will mentally rehearse. Be sure to establish clear goals for your performance.

2. *Attention to Performance Parameters*: Next, consider the "speed of movement." Re-create the exact rate of performance that is

required for successful execution of your sport. It is important to estimate how long each trial will take. This works as an indicator of your speed to completion.

3. *Attention to Kinesthetics*: Bring back the "feelings and senses" that are prevalent during movement. Develop and include cues that will facilitate your vividness and control of the imagery trial.

4. *Attention to the Environment*: Bring into your mind all those "environmental" cues that are specific to your sport and related to your performance. For example, direct attention to lane markings, yardage lines, or service lines while executing your task.

5. *Attention to Performance Cues*: Develop many positive and constructive items that will comprise the "Strategy Content." Bring into your mind words that relate to your technical performance (Knee bend, leg kick, etc.). Create all the essential performance factors and include any relevant mood words (explode off the line, rhythmic pace, etc).

6. *Attention to Success*: Establish positive and successful outcomes to your imagery trial. Establish essential performance goals and consequences of performance (e.g., winning the race and receiving a gold medal).

Focusing

The ability to focus attention immediately prior to and during performance is fundamental to achieving success. From the imaging stage, the athlete must progress away form an internal model of the performance to focusing on the external cues that are most critical for performance success. Of paramount importance is the need to release one's mind from cognitive internal rumination and shift to an external task-relevant attentional focus that prepares the body for autonomous execution. The issue for the athlete is to learn what to attend to, when to attend to it, and how to maintain that attention at the critical time.

As mentioned, attention can be conceptualized along two dimensions, breadth and direction, to account for the diverse demands of sports. Breadth refers to the amount of information the athlete attends to, while direction refers to the location of information the athlete attends to (i.e., internal versus external). As a result, an athlete's attentional style can be considered to fall within one of four possible combinations of breadth and direction at any given time (i.e., broad-external, broad-internal, narrow-external, and narrow-internal).

A broad-external focus of attention involves the processing of multiple performance cues in the sporting environment simultaneously (e.g., a quarterback scanning the defensive coverage). A broad-internal focus of attention is best suited for analyzing and integrating multiple performance cues to enhance decision making while establishing a plan of action (e.g., a pitcher deciding what pitch to throw in a given situation). A narrow-external focus of attention refers to selective attention. That is, athletes identify and attend to one or two relevant performance cues while ignoring those cues that can prove distracting (e.g., a basketball player focusing on the back of the rim just before shooting a free throw). A narrow-internal focus of attention involves the athlete identifying and attending to one or two relevant internal cues while ignoring those cues that can prove distracting, permitting the organization and mental rehearsal of performance (e.g., imaging stellar execution immediately prior to competition).

An athlete's ability to remain flexible while possessing the ability to match an attentional style to the demands of the task increases the probability for success. Attentional focus, however, extends beyond the ability to shift one's attention; it also refers to attending to one's performance. The critical notion of the focusing stage in the five-step strategy is the need for an external locus of focus on one or two critical cues at the moment of execution; directing attention outward toward task-relevant cues. This redirection of attention frees attention from explicit allocation on the plan that was developed in the imaging stage, permitting the automatic execution of the task.

One might contend that the athlete should focus his or her attention on one's own movement, adopting an internal focus. Or, should the athlete focus attention on the effects of the movement (external focus on the outcome)? Research has supported the "action effect hypothesis," which indicates that behaviors are best prepared for and executed when controlled by their intended effects, and that this can lead to enhanced performance. For example, a golfer may choose to focus on the feel and mechanics of the golf swing prior to the shot (i.e., how he or she wants to hit the ball). However, according to the action effect hypothesis, the golfer would be better served by focusing on the target and intended flight of the ball. When a skill is well learned, conscious processing of the skill merely "gets in the way," whereas attending to what the action effect would look and feel like frees the body to perform the desired action.

The focusing stage of the five-step strategy should be used by the athlete to adopt the most effective attentional strategy to meet the demands of the task. Of primary importance is to shift attention away from a conscious processing of one's actions while directing attention toward the effects of one's movement. The successful implementation of this stage seamlessly leads to the fourth stage of the five-step strategy, automatic execution.

Executing

Simply stated, this step is about letting it happen, or to borrow a phrase from Nike, "just do it!" Elite athletes perform even the most complex skills with relative ease, free from conscious thought. Being "in the zone" or operating automatically has a distinct physiological signature and has been linked to an external focus of attention (i.e., the target) as mentioned in the preceding step, rather than consciously focusing on the internal kinesthetic movements required.

The systematic observation of brain wave activity has allowed sports scientists to take a real-time look into the underlying structures of the brain that contribute to the psychological processes accounting for elite-level or expert performance. Self-paced tasks demanding hand-eye coordination, such as golf putting, archery, and marksmanship, place great demand on the attention, emotion, motor control, and preparatory systems and have proven to be instrumental for gaining insight into the psychological makeup of elite-level athletes.

The early work of sport scientists sparked a series of investigations, which examined the covert cognitive processes associated with skilled psychomotor performance of elite marksmen and other self-paced activities. To date, the majority of research in sport has relied on the decomposition of specific brain wave patterns to identify the roles of different regions of the brain in athletic performance. When comparing the left and right lobes of the brain in expert and novice performers, automaticity and cerebral efficiency were clearly evident in favor of the expert. More specifically, the expert athlete routinely demonstrated a decrease in left-brain activation with a concomitant increase or stabilization in right-brain activation. Practically speaking, these findings represent a reduction in verbal-analytic processing (self-talk) by the expert coupled with vigilant visual-spatial processing (attention to external performance cues) as the time to performance execution nears; arguably an optimal preparatory set for self-paced precision sports. Psychophysiological evidence supports the relationship between pre-performance brain specificity and the quality of performance of highly skilled participants, with greater asymmetry corresponding with increased performance. Skilled performance is optimized when conscious processing during skill execution is minimized.

In addition to the investigations into the role of the left and right hemispheres of the brain, researchers have also examined the role of slow-generating brain waves, which has provided a window to assess the activity of the brain central to the planning and initiation of voluntary movement. During target shooting, research has revealed that highly successful marksmen tend to allocate attention toward the features of the target and away from the conscious processing of the motor components of the task as indicated by the levels and location of brain activation in the few seconds immediately prior to movement execution. Conversely, suboptimal and novice performance is characterized by an attentional focus that is directed toward the requisite mechanics (i.e., gun hold) of the task in which the cortical signature during the preperformance period is denoted by a decreased readiness to act.

Research has reliably supported the notion that experts posses an extensive knowledge base that facilitates both stimulus recognition and procedural execution. Rooted in the theoretical and empirical foundation of the past 40 years devoted to understanding the attentional set of expert performance, the executing stage highlights the need to trust in the plan that is made in the imaging stage, to rely on the critical cue (s) selected during the focusing stage, and release control of executing the skill to the body that has been trained to do so.

Evaluating

The final step involves assessing the quality of task execution, outcome, and the quality of the preperformance strategy. Not unlike any skill, the preparatory routine needs to be refined and practiced frequently so that the athlete can realize the maximum benefit of engaging in such a behavior. To enhance the benefits of the preparatory routine, the athlete should systematically attend to and assess the content, implementation, and effectiveness of each component of the five-step strategy. A number of questions should be addressed when evaluating the process:

1. *What was the quality of performance?* It is important for the athlete to engage in a nonjudgmental evaluative process. That is, was the skill executed as planned, and was the outcome of the execution effective? If the quality of performance was met, it is important

to identify what was done well. If the quality of performance was not met, it is important to identify each component coupled with the required positive change.

2. *What components of the five-step strategy were helpful?* Not unlike any skill, the athlete should routinely reevaluate the contents of the five-step strategy, paying close attention to the elements that are deemed effective.

3. *What components of the five-step strategy require revision?* Where necessary, the athlete should attend to and revise ineffective components of the five-step strategy to ensure maximal benefit. Any and all changes should be systematic.

4. *What elements of the five-step strategy were planned but not executed?* The five-step strategy is a preparatory game plan that should be executed as designed. If the athlete fails to complete elements of the strategy, it is necessary to identify why. Review and identify the changes that can be made to ensure compliance.

5. *Was the optimal emotional state evoked? If not what can be done differently?* Each athlete and every skill has optimal range of emotional intensity and direction that should be experienced in order to maximize the probability for success. The athlete should take the time to attend to how they want to feel, while identifying an effective strategy for getting there.

6. *What technical/mechanical elements of the performance were executed well?* Specific skill based feedback permits positive change. It is important for athletes post competition to attend to and evaluate their technical/mechanical performance.

7. *What technical/mechanical elements of the performance could be improved? How so?* A competition debrief with a coach is an effective way to receive feedback on what changes can be made and how to go about those changes. This feedback should be constructive and free from judgment.

CONFIDENCE AND THE NEED FOR TRUST

Coaches, athletes, and sports psychologists alike support the idea that a confident athlete is more likely to be a successful athlete. If an athlete possesses the necessary skills and is sufficiently motivated to perform, the next major determinant of performance success is the belief in one's ability to achieve (i.e., self-efficacy or task specific confidence). An athlete may be the most talented, but if that athlete fails to believe in his or her ability, the superior skills they have developed will not manifest, thereby compromising performance, particularly in competition. In short, they will not realize their potential. For example a tennis player maybe be physically and technically capable of hitting a serve to close out a match, but if he or she wavers in his or her belief to execute the serve in the moment, he or she most surely will not. The critical moments immediately preceding execution must be saturate with unwavering confidence to maximize the likelihood of performance success. As such, attention is directly affected by an athlete's level of confidence. When the athlete expects success, concentration is less likely to drift to irrelevant cues spurred by self-doubt, thereby positively affecting the expectations that drive performance quality.

The application of the five-step strategy can enhance sport confidence by engaging the athlete in thought and action that is both familiar and under their direct control. During the five-step strategy, the athlete can recall successful past performances. This simple process of remembering and replaying in one's mind prior performance accomplishments can provide a momentary boost to an athlete's confidence, since that athlete is simply revisiting his or her own mastery experience; a primary source of self-efficacy.

CONCLUSIONS

Without question, appropriate attentional allocation is one of the most (if not the most) critical psychological predictors of sport performance. Since the advent of psychology, researchers have been fascinated with the concept of attention. Its multidimensional nature as well as the different attentional demands that are required for effective motor skill execution have since fascinated scientists, coaches, athletes, and even casual observers of sport competition. During the past century, a wealth of scientific, anecdotal, and experiential evidence has accumulated from which sports psychology practitioners can extract meaningful recommendations for how to best train attentional skills. This chapter has presented one approach, the five-step strategy, for understanding the multiple influences on attentional capabilities and recommendations for how to address these influences to yield optimal concentration.

While we have provided a context for the application of attention skills training and numerous examples of how such training might apply to various sport circumstances, description of the approach is intentionally broad so as to be malleable for sport-specific application.

Of critical importance is recognizing that effective attentional alloca-tion is routed in a keen awareness of the emotional, cognitive, and environmental factors that can facilitate or compromise performance. Our hope is that attentive readers will take the concepts presented herein and tailor them for application to their specific sports. Over time and with practice, recognition and awareness of critical cues can be integrated into the preperformance routine such that effortful regu-lation of attentional influences gives way to the autonomous skill exe-cution that characterizes elite athletic performance.

RECOMMENDED READING

Abernethy, B. (1988). The effects of age and expertise upon perceptual skill development in a racquet sport. *Research Quarterly for Exercise and Sport, 59*, 210–221.

Abernethy, B. (1989). Expert-novice differences in perception: How expert does the expert have to be? *Canadian Journal of Sports Sciences, 14*(1), 27–30.

Abernethy, B. (1990a). Anticipation in squash: Differences in advance cue utilization between expert and novice players. *Journal of Sports Sciences, 8*, 17–34.

Abernethy, B. (1990b). Expertise, visual search, and information pick-up in squash. *Perception, 19*, 63–77.

Abernethy, B. (1991). Visual search strategies and decision-making in sport. *International Journal of Sport Psychology, 22*, 189–210.

Abernethy, B. (1996). Training the visual-perceptual skills of athletes: Insights from the study of motor expertise. *American Journal of Sports Medicine, 24* (6), S89–S92.

Abernethy, B., Burgess-Limerick, R., & Parks, S. (1994). Contrasting approaches to the study of motor expertise. *Quest, 46*, 186–198.

Abernethy, B., & Russell, D. G. (1987a). Expert-novice differences in an applied selective attention task. *Journal of Sport Psychology, 9*, 326–345.

Abernethy, B., & Russell, D. G. (1987b). The relationship between expertise and visual search strategy in a racquet sport. *Human Movement Science, 6*, 283–319.

Abernethy, B., Neal, R. J., & Koning, P. (1994). Visual-perceptual and cognitive differences between expert, intermediate, and novice snooker players. *Applied Cognitive Psychology, 18*, 185–211.

Ainscoe, M., & Hardy, L. (1987). Cognitive warm-up in a cyclical gymnastics skill. *International Journal of Sport Psychology, 18*, 269–275.

Baddeley, A. D. (1986). *Working memory.* Oxford, UK. Clarendon Press.

Boutcher, S. H., & Crews, D. J. (1987). The effect of a preshot attentional rou-tine on a well-learned skill. *International Journal of Sport Psychology, 18*, 30–39.

Caserta, R. J., Young, J., & Janelle, C. M. (2007). Old dogs, new tricks: Training the perceptual skills of senior tennis players. *Journal of Sport and Exercise Psychology, 29*, 479–498.

Chase, W. G., & Simon, H. A. (1973). Perception in chess. *Cognitive Psychology, 4*, 55–81.

Crews, D. J. & Boutcher, S. H. (1986a). An exploratory observational analysis of professional golfers during competition. *Journal of Sport Behavior, 9*, 51–58.

Crews, D. J. & Boutcher, S. H. (1986b). Effects of structured preshot behaviors on beginning golf performance. *Perceptual and Motor Skills, 62*, 291–294.

Davidson, R. J. (2004). What does the prefrontal cortex "do" in affect: perspectives on EEG frontal asymmetry research. *Biological Psychology, 67*, 219–233.

Deeny, S., Hillman, C. H., Janelle, C. M., & Hatfield, B. D. (2003). Cortico-cortical communication and superior performance in skilled marksman: An EEG coherence analysis. *Journal of Exercise and Sport Psychology, 25*, 188–204.

Easterbrook, E. A. (1959). The effect of emotion on cue utilization and the organization of behavior. *Psychological Review, 66*(3), 183–201.

Edmonds, W. A., Mann, D. T. Y., Tennenbaum, G., & Janelle, C. M. (2006). Analysis of affect related performance zones: An idiographic approach using psychophysiological and introspective data. *Sport Psychologist, 20*, 40–57.

Eysenck, M. W., & Calvo, M. G. (1992). Anxiety and performance: The processing efficiency theory. *Cognition and Emotion, 6*(6), 409–434.

Hanin, Y. (2007). Emotions in sport: Current issues and perspectives. In G. Tenenbaum & R. C. Eklund (Eds.), *Handbook of sport psychology* (3rd ed., pp. 31–58). Hoboken, NJ: John Wiley & Sons, Inc.

Hanton, S., & Jones, G. (1999). The effects of a multimodal intervention program on performers: II. Training the butterflies to fly in formation. *Sport Psychologist, 13*, 22–41.

Hardy, L., & Callow, N. (1999). Efficacy of external and internal visual imagery perspectives for the enhancement of performance on tasks in which form is important. *Journal of Sport and Exercise Psychology, 21*, 95–112.

Hatfield, B. D., Haufler, A. J., Hung, T. M., & Spalding, T. W. (2004). Electroencephalographic (EEG) studies of skilled psychomotor performance. *Clinical Neurophysiology, 21*, 144–156.

Hatfield, B. D., Landers, D. M., & Ray, W. J. (1984). Cognitive processes during self-paced motor performance: An electroencephalographic profile of skilled marksmen. *Journal of Sport Psychology, 6*, 42–59.

Hatfield, B. D., Landers, D. M., & Ray, W. J. (1987). Cardiovascular-CNS interactions during a self-paced, intentional attentive state. Elite marksmanship performance. *Psychophysiology, 24*, 542–549.

Hatfield, B. D., Landers, D. M., Ray, W. J., & Daniels, F. S. (1982). An electroencephalographic study of elite rifle shooters. *The American Marksman, 7*, 6–8.

Jacobson, E. (1930). Electrical measurements of neuromuscular states during mental activities. I. *American Journal of Physiology, 91*, 547–608.

Jacobson, E. (1932). Muscular phenomenon during imagining. *American Journal of Psychology, 49*, 677–694.

Janelle, C. M. (2002). Anxiety, arousal and visual attention: A mechanistic account of performance variability. *Journal of Sports Sciences, 20*, 237–251.

Janelle, C. M., & Hatfield, B. (2008). Visual attention and brain processes that underlie expert performance: Implications for sport and military psychology. *Military Psychology, 20*, 117–134.

Janelle, C. M., & Hillman, C. H. (2003). Expert performance in sport: Current perspective and critical issues. In J. L. Starkes & K. A. Erikson (Eds). *Expert performance in sports: Advances in research on sport expertise* (pp. 19–48). Champaign, IL: Human Kinetics.

Janelle, C. M., Hillman, C. H., Apparies, R. J., Murray, N. P., Meili, L., Fallon, E. A., & Hatfield, B. D. (2000). Expertise differences in cortical activation and gaze behavior during rifle shooting. *Journal of Sport and Exercise Psychology, 22*, 167–182.

Janelle, C. M., Hillman, C. H., & Hatfield, B.D. (2000). Concurrent measurement of electroencephalographic and ocular indices of attention during rifle shooting: An exploratory case study. *International Journal of Sports Vision, 6*(1), 21–29.

Janelle, C. M., Singer, R. N., & Williams, A. M. (1999). External distraction and attentional narrowing: Visual search evidence. *Journal of Sport and Exercise Psychology, 21* (1), 70–91.

Jasper, H. H. (1958). Report of the committee on methods of clinical examination in electroencephalography. *Journal of Electroencephalography and Clinical Neurophysiology, 10*, 370–375.

Jones, C., & Miles, J. (1978). Use of advance cues in predicting the flight of a lawn tennis ball. *Journal of Human Movement Studies, 4*, 231–235.

Jones, G., & Swain, A. B. J. (1992). Intensity and direction dimensions of competitive state anxiety and relationships with competitiveness. *Perceptual and Motor Skills, 74*, 467–472.

Kerick, S. E., Douglass, L., & Hatfield, B. D. (2004). Cerebral cortical adaptations associated with visuomotor practice. *Medicine & Science in Sport and Exercise, 36*, 118–129.

Konttinen, N., Landers, D. M., & Lyytinen, H. (2000). Aiming routines and their electrocortical concomitants among competitive rifle shooters. *Scandinavian Journal of Medicine & Science in Sports, 10* (3), 169–177.

Konttinen, N., Lyytinen, H., & Era, P. (1999). Brain slow potentials and postural sway behavior during sharpshooting performance. *Journal of Motor Behavior, 31*, 11–20.

Konttinen, N., & Lyytinen, H., & Konttinen, R. (1995). Brain slow potentials reflecting successful shooting performance. *Research Quarterly for Exercise and Sport, 66*, 64–72.

Lerner, B. S., Ostrow, A. C., Yura, M. T., & Etzel, E. F. (1996). The effects of goal-setting and imagery training programs on the free-throw performance of female collegiate basketball players. *Sport Psychologist, 10,* 382–397.

Liebert, R. M., & Morris, L. W. (1967). Cognitive and emotional components of test anxiety: A distinction and some initial data. *Psychological Reports, 20,* 975–978.

Mann, D. T. Y., William, A. M., Ward, P., & Janelle, C. M. (2006). Perceptual-cognitive expertise in sport: A meta-analysis. *Journal of Sport and Exercise Psychology, 29,* 457–478.

Masters, R. S. W. (1992). Knowledge, knerves and know-how: The role of explicit versus implicit knowledge in the breakdown of a complex motor skull under pressure. *British Journal of Psychology, 83,* 343–358.

Moran, A. P. (1996). *The psychology of concentration in sport performers.* East Sussex, UK: Psychology Press.

Murray, N. M., & Janelle, C. M. (2003). Anxiety and performance: A visual search examination of the processing efficiency theory. *Journal of Sport and Exercise Psychology, 25,* 171–187.

Murray, N. P., & Janelle, C. M. (2007). Event-related potential evidence for the processing efficiency theory. *Journal of Sports Sciences, 25,* 161–171.

Nideffer, R. M. (1985). *An athletes' guide to mental training.* Champaign, IL: Human Kinetics.

Orlick, T., & Partington, J. (1988). Mental links to excellence. *Sport Psychologist, 2,* 105–130.

Patrick, T. D., & Hrycaiko, D. W. (1998). Effects of a mental training package on an endurance performance. *Sport Psychologist, 12,* 283–299.

Predebon, J., & Docker, S. B. (1992). Free-throw shooting performance as a function of preshot routines. *Perceptual and Motor Skills, 75,* 167–171.

Richman, H. B., Gobet, F., Staszewski, J. J., & Simon, H. A. (1996). Perceptual and memory processes in the acquisition of expert performance. In K. A. Ericsson (Ed.), *The road to excellence: The acquisition of expert performance in the arts and sciences, sports, and games* (pp.167–187). Mahwah, NJ: Lawrence Erlbaum Associates.

Richardson, A. (1969). *Mental imagery.* New York: Springer Publishing Company, Inc.

Rushall, B. S. (1970). Some application of psychology to swimming. *Swimming Technique, 7,* 71–82.

Rushall, B. S. (1995). *Mental skills training for sports.* Spring Valley, CA: Sports Science Associates.

Rushall, B. S., & Lippman, L. G. (1998). The role of imagery in physical performance. *International Journal of Sport Psychology, 29,* 57–72.

Sackett, R. S. (1934). The influences of symbolic rehearsal upon the retention of a maze habit. *Journal of General Psychology, 13,* 113–128.

Schneider, W., & Chein, J. M. (2003). Controlled and automatic processing: behavior, theory, and biological mechanisms. *Cognitive Science, 27,* 525–559.

Singer, R. N. (1988). Strategies and metastrategies in learning and performing self-paced athletic skills. *Sport Psychologist, 2*, 49–68.

Singer, R. N., & Janelle, C. M. (1999). Determining sport expertise: From genes to supremes. *International Journal of Sport Psychology, 30*, 117–150.

Singer, R. N., Lidor, R., & Cauraugh, J. H. (1993). To be aware of not aware? What to think about while learning and performing a motor skill. *Sport Psychologist, 7*, 19–30.

Suinn, R. M. (1972). Behavior rehearsal training for skiers. *Behavior Therapy, 3*, 210–221.

Williams, A. M., & Elliot, D. (1999). Anxiety, expertise and visual search strategy in karate. *Journal of Sport & Exercise Psychology, 21*, 361–374.

Williams, A. M, Singer, R., & Frehlich, S. (2002). Quiet eye duration, expertise, and task complexity in near and far aiming tasks. *Journal of Motor Behavior, 34*, 197–207.

Williams, M. A., Vickers, J., & Rodrigues, S. (2002). The effects of anxiety on visual search, movement kinematics, and performance in table tennis: A test of Eysenck and Calvo's processing efficiency theory. *Journal of Sport & Exercise Psychology, 24*(4), 438–455.

Woolfolk, R. L., Parrish, M. W., & Murphy, S. M. (1985). The effects of positive and negative imagery on motor skill performance. *Cognitive Therapy and Research, 9*, 335–341.

Wrisberg, C. A. & Pein, R. L. (1992). The preshot interval and free throw accuracy: An exploratory investigation. *Sport Psychologist, 6*, 14–23.

Wulf, G., & Shea, C. H. (2002). Principles derived from the study of simple skills do not generalize to complex skill learning. *Psychonomic Bulletin & Review, 9*(2), 185–211.

Chapter 3

Psychosocial Aspects of Coaching and Leadership

Ralph A. Vernacchia

The interrelationship of athletic coaching behaviors, strategies, tech-niques, and leadership skills is both multifaceted and critical in terms of determining the quality and effectiveness of the sport experience for athletes at all levels of participation. Coaching can be viewed as a subset of leadership, especially when one considers that the coach is responsible for developing not only athletic talent, but also the train-ing and performance climate that fosters the healthy pursuit of athletic excellence.

It should be noted that from a historical perspective, the psychology of coaching gave impetus to the emergence of sport psychology as a viable sport science in the late 1950s, 1960s, and early 1970s. Early texts regarding the relationship and influence of psychology on coaching effectiveness and athletic performance were embraced by physical educators and coaches and, in many ways, the psychology of coaching continues to be a "best fit" for the principles of contemporary applied sports psychology.

This chapter will explore the psychosocial aspects of coaching and athletic leadership, including the world of the coach, the influence of the coach, athletic leadership, the cornerstones of effective coaching, and holistic coaching. Each of these aspects of effective coaching plays an important and integral role in the development of both athletic talent and personal excellence.

THE WORLD OF THE COACH

Coaches realize that they are often expected to be "all things to all people" and consequently are required to maintain a flexible leadership role with the athletes they coach and, in some cases, the parents of the athletes they coach. Coaches are oftentimes surrogate parents, mentors, teachers, administrators, friends, etc., to the athletes they coach. Most importantly, coaches are teachers of sport who are expected and trusted to safeguard and perpetuate programs that provide quality educational experiences for each athlete at various developmental levels (youth, high school, college/university, club). As a result of their involvement in the athletic world, coaches may experience and derive a great deal of satisfaction and fulfillment from the influential role they play in the lives of the athletes they coach.

Coaches, especially at the elite and professional levels, live in a "fish-bowl" world of absolutes: winning and losing. Every move they make, particularly when related to performance outcomes or effectiveness, is clearly visible to those around them. Many coaches experience a sense of urgency created by the heightened expectations of the media, alumni, fans, parents, etc., and the ever-present judgment that "you are only as good as your last game or season." The reality of athletic achievement motivation is that no matter how well you do, it is never quite good enough. The coach who wins a championship is expected to win again next year; and if the coach wins two or three championships in a narrow time frame, demands for a "dynasty" increase performance expectations and coaching pressures. This is the coaching challenge of athletic leadership that can exist in a world of forced achievement and unrealistic expectations.

In the coach's world, professional advancement and job security often depend on the performance of young and inexperienced athletes, over whom the coach has little control once the athletic contest begins. In addition, coaches are involved in a profession that is not very cost effective. In fact, for many coaches, coaching is only a part of what they do for a living. Many are considered part-time or even serve as volunteer coaches. Coaching responsibilities are often layered upon existing job and family responsibilities, which contributes to coaching stress in the form of role conflict or role strain.

For example, one of the most common role conflict or role strain situations occurs if coaches are also schoolteachers. The demands of serving in both these roles can be overwhelming as they prepare for classes each day, grade exams and assignments, manage classroom behaviors, teach a number of classes each day, and then prepare for conducting practice sessions, attend to the needs of student-athletes, travel to competitions, manage budgets, facilities, and equipment, coach their teams, interact with parents, administrators, and the media, and more. Add to this the possible coach and family conflicts and strain that coaches often experience, and it is easy to see why coaches are often labeled as "stress seekers" who often raise everyone else's children but their own.

Although there are some high-profile coaches who are handsomely rewarded for their efforts and accomplishments, most coaches toil in a world that values their going to work early and coming home late, regardless of financial compensation. For most coaches, salaries and fringe benefits are low or nonexistent, and work time demands are high. The bottom line for many coaches is that they are often under-resourced and overworked as they pursue their love of sport and passion for coaching.

THE INFLUENCE OF THE COACH

Leadership in general can be defined as the one's ability to influence others to do things well. Given this definition, coaches certainly have the opportunity to play an influential role in the lives of the athletes they coach. Coaches spend a considerable amount of time with the athletes who are members of the teams they coach and the programs they oversee. However, coaching effectiveness is determined by the coaches' ability to influence others to do certain things well. Coaching effectiveness is often determined by the coach's ability to understand and implement the philosophical, ethical, and scientific foundations of athletic performance.

The athlete meets sport at the coach, and therefore, the educational quality of the athletic experience for each athlete is determined, in large part, by the philosophical and ethical orientation of the coach. The coach provides the leadership, guidance, and authority to make the athletic experience and educational meaningful and fulfilling for each athlete. Philosophically, for example, a coach may, select the theme of "coach the person first, and the sport second" to guide their team values and orientation in recognition of the critical influence that a coach can have on the physical, emotional, ethical, and social development of an athlete. Unfortunately, on the other side of the coaching philosophy continuum is the "win at all costs" coaching orientation that encourages false sport ethics such as "the ends justify the means." The ethical orientation of the coach will ultimately determine each coach's leadership style and coaching philosophy.

The values and foundational beliefs of an athletic program can provide the guidance for administrators, coaches, athletes, and parents to consistently follow and implement throughout the sport season. For example, one foundational belief statement and objective that guides coaching behavior could be "the development of self-confidence through the use of one's own decision-making capabilities." This statement emphasizes the ability of sport to build confidence if athletes are allowed to make decisions for themselves, by themselves, and about themselves. Furthermore, programmatic goals can emphasize the promotion of sportspersonship and character development by emphasizing team and individual themes such as "athletic excellence with integrity" and "winning is important, but it is not the only thing; character counts."

Coaches are well served to define and express their coaching philosophy and team goals, policies, and guidelines or rules in a parent-coach meeting that can be held at the beginning of each season. Such a meeting can only foster parental support that can enhance team unity and performance while at the same time establishing clearly defined team and individual standards and behaviors. In addition, developing a team handbook that defines the team's philosophy, goals, policies, standards, and values, as well as many of the operational dimensions of the team (scheduling, facilities and equipment access, practice procedures, travel procedures, etc.), can be an essential educational team resource that can promote coach-athlete-parent communication and team unity.

It is also essential that coaches have a working knowledge of the sport sciences as a foundation for their qualifications and competencies to coach. Basic foundations of sport science, including growth and development, exercise physiology, biomechanics, sports psychology, nutrition, strength training, etc., can be acquired through formal education (kinesiology, exercise, and sport science or physical education degree) or through a variety of coaching education programs that are available to coaches.

Sports psychology professionals Greg Dale and Jeff Janssen have identified and defined the characteristics of highly credible coaches as character, competency, commitment, caring, being a confidence builder, communication, and consistency. Each of these characteristics or desirable coaching traits are linked to coaching success and emphasize the importance of leadership as a key component in determining whether athletes reach their personal and athletic potential.

Dale encourages coaches to develop these characteristics by pursuing the following behavioral goals: tell the truth and emphasize character with athletes (character); as a coach, be inquisitive and innovative (competency); practice what you preach and teach, live your passion and vision (commitment); make the athletes whom you coach your priority (caring); communicate belief in each athlete's ability to reach their performance potential (confidence builder); master effective communication techniques and the ability to communicate athletic performance knowledge to each athlete (communication); and be consistent in the application of accountability of team rules and expectations (consistency).

COACHING AND ATHLETIC LEADERSHIP

Essential to the understanding of the principles of effective athletic leadership is the ability of the coach to separate leadership responsibilities from managerial duties. There are many managerial tasks that coaches perform on a daily basis that are critical to the success of their programs (i.e., budgeting, recruiting, staffing, ordering equipment, fund-raising, scheduling, travel arrangements, etc.). The adage that "you manage things and lead people" can go a long way in helping coaches focus of the essentials of athletic leadership.

A formula that illustrates the components of athletic leadership is:

$$
\begin{aligned}
\text{Leadership} = \ &\text{Integrity} \times \text{Communication} \\
&\times \text{Understanding of Human Behavior} \\
&\times \text{Knowledge of Sport}
\end{aligned}
$$

Integrity

Paramount to the coach's leadership success is the development and maintenance of a trusting relationship with each team member, which ensures that individuals will be treated fairly. The coach's power as a leader is derived from two factors: position and trust. It is not enough to have the title "coach." Coaches endeavor to earn the respect and loyalty of each team member through honest and sincere daily interactions. These interactions occur in a cooperative and competitive environment of athletic participation that continually presents opportunities for personal growth as well as performance excellence.

Communication

A coach's vision or programmatic goals are only ideological. They become real once the coach is able to clearly and understandably communicate the team vision and goals to team members through the process of "intellectual persuasion." The effectiveness of any team or individual team member to achieve program and personal goals is dependant upon the athlete's ability to understand, accept, and actualize team philosophy, standards, norms, and goals.

Understanding of Human Behavior

Coaching psychology is all about understanding the motivations and actions of athletic performers. Effective coaches understand the physical, mental, emotional, and social dynamics that underlie and influence the behavior and performance outcomes of the athletes they coach. Leaders who have empathy and can relate compassionately with their followers can provide the social support, encouragement, insights, feedback, and incentives necessary for an athlete's personal improvement and self-actualization.

Knowledge of Sport

Athletes seek experts or knowledgeable leaders who are educated, trained, and experienced in the art and science of athletic performance. Athletes choose a coach who has the sport-specific knowledge and experience necessary to help them realize their athletic dream. The coach is then charged with the responsibility of knowing people (human behavior) and knowing sport (training and performance strategies and techniques) while providing the guidance and feedback necessary to enable athletes to realize their performance goals.

THE COACH'S LEADERSHIP STYLE

The coach's ability to communicate and influence team members is directly related to his or her leadership style. Essentially, coaches can choose to be task-oriented or people-oriented leaders of their teams. As a result of the performance demands involved in coaching athletic teams, the majority of coaches tend to adopt a task-oriented leadership style that is purposeful and directive.

A task-oriented coaching style can be either autocratic or dictatorial in its communication and interaction orientations. An autocratic coaching style is characterized by a one-way communication pattern that flows from the coach to the athlete and/or team. This style is sometimes referred to as the "my way or the highway" approach to coaching, and the team members are oriented to the programmatic goals of the coach.

A dictatorial coaching style provides more communication flexibility between the coach and athlete. In this style, there is a two-way communication between the athlete and/or team members, but the coach has the final say in all team matters and performance-related decisions.

The advantages of using a task-oriented leadership style (autocratic or dictatorial) are that this coaching style: is more efficient, with energy directed primarily toward the task; requires little time taken for interpersonal communication; enables coaches to designate jobs quickly in highly structured task situations; is effective in situations highly favorable to leadership (i.e., high leader power and obvious task requirements); and enables the coach to be effective in highly unfavorable situations (i.e., low leader power, unstructured task, or resistant group members).

The disadvantages of a task-oriented leadership style (autocratic or dictatorial) are that this coaching style: may raise anxiety levels of certain group members in response to the command-response style of the coach or lack of athlete input on team, practice, and performance decisions; sacrifices the personal security of team members for expediency, since athletes are expected to execute the directions of the coaches oftentimes without discussion or questioning; is less effective in moderately stressful situations in which team members may wish to interact; and may not work well with key team members who have a need for serving in a leadership role, such as a team captain.

A word of caution is appropriate here for the task-oriented coach who elects to use an autocratic leadership style. Oftentimes autocratic coaches use punishment to deter and correct performance errors and personal behaviors of their athletes. Punishment or negative reinforcement will tend to create a "fear of failure" orientation in athletes, resulting in a tendency for team members to play conservatively in an effort to avoid making mistakes and consequently being singled out or punished by the coach. Seasoned coaches learn to "praise in public and criticize in private," thus avoiding embarrassing athletes in front of their teammates, friends, family, the media, and fans. Constructive evaluations using positive reinforcement and instructive feedback can be extremely effective in helping athletes master the daily performance challenges that are presented in various practice and competitive situations.

The punishment or negative approach to coaching is detrimental to an athlete's performance because mistakes are an integral part of athletic participation and contests. In fact, the most successful athletes learn that sports are games of mistakes; effective athletic performances are not about making mistakes, but it is what you do after you make a mistake that really counts. The athlete who can be taught to accept and learn from their mistakes will, in the long run, be more effective, since they are willing to respond to performance challenges and outcomes in a way that combines effort and skill effectively in challenging and risky competitive situations.

This is not to say that autocratic coaches are unsuccessful in the athletic world. Many task-oriented leaders are highly successful coaches primarily because they understand the delicate balance between positive and negative reinforcement in establishing leadership power and effectiveness. Essentially, the leader's power and effectiveness is dependent upon: (1) how the leader uses authority, and (2) the ability to gain the respect and trust of followers. Coaches can enhance their power by not only encouraging their athletes to strive for realistic and quality performance standards, but also by demonstrating a sincere concern for their athletes' welfare, both on and off the athletic field.

People-oriented coaches are social leaders whose leadership style can be characterized as either democratic or laissez-faire. A democratic leadership style provides an atmosphere of "equal say" between the coach and athlete and/or team. Each team member, including the coach, contributes equally to team decisions and policies. Decisions in this type of leadership style are made by consensus.

A laissez-faire or "do as you please" leadership style is characterized by mixed communication between the coach and the team members. In this "anything goes" style of leadership, the coach serves in more a managerial role, similar to coaches at the professional sport levels. Individuality is the norm when this type of leadership style is employed by the coach.

Advantages of a people-oriented or social leadership style (democratic or laissez-faire) include: it may reduce athlete tension and worries in situations when teams lose or individuals fail; it can help the coach be more responsive to insecure people by utilizing a two-way communication flow between the coach and athlete, thus allowing for athlete input and opportunities to express concerns about performance outcomes; it can help the coach perform more effectively in challenging situations and provides a mechanism for shared decision making between coach and athlete; and it is most appropriate with teams and athletes who are more mature and experienced.

The disadvantages of a people-oriented or social leadership style (democratic or laissez-faire) include: there can be a lack of concern about successful execution of the task; the coach is less effective in highly stressful situations or those in which great power or power symbols are obviously awarded to the coach; and this style may cause anxious responses in team members who are highly task-oriented.

TEAM DYNAMICS

Once the educational philosophy of an athletic program is developed and clearly communicated by the coach, a team will typically progress through four stages in its development. These stages are: Forming, Storming, Norming, and Performing. This popular model has been used by sports psychologists to explain the group process in sport in an effort to enhance and facilitate the two most essential interrelated components of this process, namely, communication and productivity (see Table 3.1).

Forming

The initial, forming stage, involves the process of team selection, which is a nervous time for the athlete. Their skills and talents are under close scrutiny and constant evaluation. This is a time of intense intra-team competition, personal anxiety, and uncertainty for all players. Veteran players may perceive new recruits as a threat to their formerly secure positions on the team.

Once the team is selected, it becomes essential for the coach to clarify and explain each player's role and responsibilities. Program standards and the philosophy, purpose, and mission of the program should also be clearly communicated and defined by the coaching staff.

It is also during this stage that team goals and individual goals are formulated. This can be accomplished in a variety of ways, but the coach must decide whether goals are to be leader-formulated or team-formulated, or whether the coaching staff and the team will share responsibility for formulated goals. It should be noted that if the team is involved in the formulation of team goals, they will be more likely to behave in ways that will help them realize these goals.

Table 3.1
Team-building Stages and Characteristics

Team-building Stage	Stage Characteristics
Forming	• Team selection • Nervous time • Roles explained, clarified, and assigned • Goals set • Belief in program standards • Commitment to program standards and goals • Trust, acceptance, and concern/care for teammates
Storming	• The stage of role acceptance • Conflicts as a result of miscommunication and misinterpretation, "scoreboard mentality," close quarters, individual differences in lifestyle and behavior • Conflict resolution • Recommitment to program standards and goals
Norming	• Stage of role performance • Group accepts and feels comfortable with their roles and responsibilities • Teamwork evident—team members openly support and encourage each other
Performing	• Stage of role maintenance • The artistic and creative stage • The flow stage • Silent communication and understanding between players • This stage is not self-sustaining; you may have to return to the storming stage and rebuild

It is also advisable for teams to set both *product* and *process* goals. Most teams are very concerned with product or outcome goals and neglect the process goals, which have a considerable impact on players' enjoyment of the athletic experience. A common product or outcome goal of a team is to "win." A process goal that accompanies winning would be to become fit and healthy through participation in practice sessions.

Once team selection has taken place and roles and goals have been identified, the team will begin to establish team social norms that will govern the behavior of the group members. A team identity is formed, and a trusting team environment is established that stresses acceptance and sincere concern and care for teammates.

Belief in and commitment to the program standards and goals are expected to supersede individual performance goals during the forming stage, and cooperative behaviors (teamwork) are encouraged in an effort to attain team success. This is especially important in highly interactive and interdependent sports such as football, basketball, soccer, and volleyball.

Storming

A familiar quote that best describes this stage is: "A ship is safe in the harbor, but that's not what it's built for." Conflict is a natural and healthy part of the group process. Specific suggestions for dealing effectively with conflict (conflict resolution methods) will be presented later, but the essential point is that conflict must be addressed and dealt with expeditiously and in accordance with previously established program standards and group norms. If not dealt with in this manner, conflicts and disagreements can rapidly erode team morale and cohesion.

Conflict within athletic teams usually results from the inability and unwillingness of certain individuals to accept their assigned roles or the team standards, norms, and goals. Other sources of team conflict are: athlete-athlete or coach-athlete miscommunication; misinterpretation of team policies; scoreboard mentality (emphasis on individual goals at the expense of teamwork and group success); overexposure to the same individuals in an intense training, traveling, and competitive environment; and an intolerance of idiosyncrasies of team members.

Once conflict is resolved, the group or individuals involved recommits to the program standards and team goals. If not handled properly, a team may remain in the storming stage and eventually become unproductive.

Norming

Once the group members have accepted their roles and understand the relationship of these roles to overall group performance, the group can begin to function as a team. In this stage, each member in the group fulfills the responsibilities of his or her assigned roles. Teamwork becomes evident in this stage as team members openly support and encourage each other.

Performing

This phase of team development is often referred to as the "flow stage." At this stage, accepted roles are maintained as the team artistically, creatively, and effectively accomplishes its goals. There is an unspoken understanding between team members as well as between the coach and the team members. The coach should take care to maintain this stage since a return to the storming stage would require that the rebuilding process begin anew.

COHESION AND TEAM BUILDING

Task Cohesion and Mastery

The training and practice patterns of team members requires a tremendous commitment to task cohesion—that is, toward the mastery of physical conditioning and motor skill development that will ultimately result in effective individual performance within the team context. Mastering the execution and performance of movement skills in challenging competitive situations is the key to athletic performance in any sport.

Effective athletic performances result from taking one's ability and improving it through conscientious practice until it is equal to meet the demands of the performance setting. Once an athlete can master their event and meet the demands of competition, sport becomes more enjoyable as the athlete becomes proud of their preparation and ability to reach team and personal performance goals. Individual pride as a result of hard work and task or event mastery can form a sense of collective competency among team members as they view their ability to undertake performance challenges.

Coaches can promote and target task cohesion by promoting quality practice or training efforts. By engaging in quality practice sessions, rather than merely going through the motions at practice, athletes can develop a shared sense of pride in both their team and individual work ethic and accomplishments. Remember, we play like we practice, so in order to engage in quality practice sessions, athletes should practice with a purpose (know why they are doing certain practice drills and training activities, such as strength-training exercises), set clear daily goals for practice (most athletes set goals for the game, very few set goals for each day's practice session), and engage, with help from the coaching staff, in constructive evaluation of each practice session.

Social Cohesion

Team-building activities that develop social cohesion are important in any sport because they provide opportunities for team members to interact with each other. These activities can include team meals, team social gatherings and activities, team travel, as well as training activities such as group runs, group warm-ups, and team stretching and flexibility.

Most importantly, team activities designed to build social cohesion set the stage for generating the social support necessary to succeed in demanding training and performance settings. Practicing in isolation, training in various climatic conditions, injuries, poor performances or performance slumps, and balancing life and academic demands are but a few of the occurrences that can ultimately influence and interfere with the attainment of team and personal performance goals.

SOCIAL SUPPORT AND TEAM-BUILDING

Social support strategies can facilitate the team-building process by providing team members with opportunities for social and emotional growth within the demanding context of the athletic arena. These strategies and activities can be helpful in the team-building process by promoting communication among team members, and between team members and the coach, which in turn provides team members with a sense of physical and mental well-being, and satisfaction with team experiences and leadership. As an intervention strategy, social support can provide the encouragement and resources necessary to reduce stress, combat overtraining and burnout, increase feelings of well-being, and overcome feelings of isolation associated with training.

Support, encouragement, care, and concern provided by teammates and coaches are essential in providing the motivational fuel necessary to overcome adversity and to provide meaning for an athlete's quest for performance excellence. Social support strategies and activities are specifically helpful in developing communication among team member and between coaches and athletes, which, in turn, can lead to a shared team vision and commitment to team goals and values.

The following social support techniques and strategies can be utilized in the team building process:

Listening Support: Team members feel someone can listen to their concerns and problems without giving advice and being judgmental. Listening support is characterized by nonjudgmental active listening between team members and team staff regarding the stress of training and performance demands; providing group social events for coaches, staff, and athletes so they can "step out of sport" and their roles within the team and relate to each other on a more personal level; promote informal contacts between team members, the coaching staff, and other support personnel; and structure the practice environment to convey warmth, friendliness, and acceptance.

Emotional Support: Team members are provided with a feeling of care and concern, that someone is on their side. This aspect of social support is characterized by the importance of emotional support to team leaders so they may provide and model such support for team members; encourage emotional support for injured athletes; encourage the staff to be available to team members away from practice; make the services of a sports psychology professional available to the team and staff.

Emotional Challenge Support: Team members feel that others challenge them to evaluate their attitudes, values, and feelings. This type of social support is provided by friends, parents, and coaches, not teammates; use of team meetings, team talks, and team themes, etc. to help team members focus, or in some cases, refocus their emotional energy on their performance; teammates provide verbal encouragement in challenging training and performance situations.

Task Appreciation Support: Team members and coaches acknowledge the efforts of teammates and promote an appreciation for team and individual work ethic. Team members and coaches reinforce and affirm the training effort of teammates who are striving to master their event skills through conscientious and dedicated practice; provide awards ceremonies that reward improvement as well as outstanding performances; and use the media to convey the value and significance of performance accomplishments.

Task Challenge Support: Team members are made to feel that others will challenge them to challenge themselves in terms of improving their ability and performance effectiveness. Coaches and teammates can provide positive reinforcement and information/corrective feedback to challenge athletes to enhance training and performance efforts; use of technology (i.e., visual digital recordings, etc.) to provide feedback and enhance performance; athletes are encouraged to accept task challenge as a team responsibility and norm.

Tangible Assistance Support: This type of social support provides resources such as training equipment and facilities, economic support (i.e., scholarships, per diem, etc.), and travel to competitions.

Personal Assistance Support: This type of social support provides team members with lifestyle support, and teammates help each other with academic interests (peer advising), transportation to social events, errands, personal needs during injury rehabilitation, etc.

CORNERSTONES OF EFFECTIVE COACHING AND ATHLETIC LEADERSHIP

Anticipation, preparation, communication and dedication are the cornerstones of effective coaching. Coaches pride themselves on their ability to mentally, physically, emotionally, and, in some cases, spiritually prepare their teams and athletes for competitive performances. To this end, coaches dedicate themselves to anticipating the numerous competitive challenges that may be experienced by the teams and athletes they coach.

Anticipation and Preparation

Anticipation and preparation are the keys to mental toughness. The ability and intent to perform in a non-distractible way with a clear and present focus often separates the contenders from the pretenders and the also-rans when it comes to delivering effective athletic performances.

Coaches are mindful that they must "expect the unexpected" if they are going to mentally and physically prepare their athletes to perform effectively in athletic competition. Coaches do all possible to address the "what ifs" of athletic performance by teaching athletes how to develop and implement mental and physical contingency plans that will serve them well in the face of adversity.

Common mental training techniques that can be employed by athletes to facilitate this process are mental rehearsal and concentration strategies such as visualization, attuning, relaxation training, creative concentration, mental routines, and distraction control training. Sports psychology professionals often remind athletes, for example, that effective athletic performance is not determined by one's ability to focus, but by one's ability to refocus.

Communication

The ability of the coach to effectively communicate and demonstrate the ideas and philosophy regarding the team's mission and goals is an essential prerequisite for the team-building process and, ultimately, for the team's success. As stated previously, athletes seek the security of fairness, care, and concern in the team environment, and the coach is the gatekeeper of the team process. The coach must be able to communicate, through word and action, his or her care, concern, and support for the each athlete's committed training and performance efforts. Rick McGuire, head track and field coach at the University of Missouri and a sports psychology professional, has suggested the following basic communication guidelines for enhancing the team building process:

1. Always communicate with those below you as you would wish to be communicated with by those from above you! This is no more than the "Golden Rule" applied to issues of communication within a team.
2. Seek to have important communications within a team be provided in a REGULAR, CONSISTENT, and THOROUGH manner.
3. Always take care of the "Bottom Rung."

Coach-athlete communication can always take place in a respectful way, a way that emphasizes the positive and provides feedback to improve on the negative. It is essential that throughout this process, coaches remind athletes that any feedback that they might provide is about the athlete's performance or behavior and not about the athlete personally. This friendly reminder is helpful in creating an open communication atmosphere between coach and athlete based on constructive feedback.

Coaches can use the "sandwich approach" to provide constructive feedback in sports. Essentially, this approach begins by providing the athlete with a positive statement regarding his or her training or performance efforts and then providing the corrective, informative, or prescriptive feedback necessary to successfully perform a specific skill or behavior in the future. In the final stage of this approach, the coach compliments the athlete on the improvement he or she has made and encourages the athlete to sustain his or her efforts until the performance skill or behavior is mastered.

Since conflict is a "natural" part of the team-building process (the storming stage), it is also important for coaches and athletes to be trained in conflict resolution methods. Intra-team conflicts usually stem from miscommunication and misinterpretation of team standards, norms, roles, and goals—how the coaching staff and team members respond to intra-team conflict can make or break a team. Coaches and athletes can learn that intra-team conflicts (coach-athlete, athlete-athlete) are a natural part of the team-building process if addressed respectfully and expeditiously in a climate of respect.

Dedication

In general, coaches are highly motivated individuals who are dedicated to their profession. They tend to be altruistic leaders who often overwork in an attempt to motivate their athletes to consistently perform at the highest levels. The major professional issue for contemporary coaches at all levels is not dedication, but overdedication. The athletic world, with its emphasis on achievement, rewards, recognition, and status, provide fertile ground to cultivate coaches who soon become immersed in the culture of the over-motivated underachiever. This is a culture that transforms energetic and enthusiastic coaches into exhausted individuals who are "just too tired to care about anything in their lives."

Coaches are also on an occupational merry-go-round that is difficult to leave. Athletes come and go. For those coaches who remain, the year-to-year accumulation of job-related stress becomes increasingly burdensome. In addition, college and high school coaches may be faced with a generation gap that develops between themselves and their athletes. Coaches get older, but their athletes remain at the same age and developmental level. As a result, coaches may find that there are important differences between their interests and those of young athletes. Although coaches emphasize being focused on athletic performance, many of today's young athletes find it difficult to stay focused on one task. Patience can wear thin for focus-oriented coaches who demand and expect undivided attention to the ways, means, and objectives of athletic training and performance.

In addition, this is the age of the technocoach. Advances in the sport sciences and technology have served to encourage overcoaching and over-preparation of athletes for competition. The availability of computers, video and digital cameras, rehabilitative methodologies and equipment, and nutritional supplementation, coupled with the proliferation of performance enriching information and training methods, place an inordinate demand on coaches to keep up with the latest developments in their sport. The challenge for contemporary coaches is to maintain their feel for the art of coaching while at the same time mastering the science of their sport.

It is over-dedication that can often produce unhealthy levels of coaching stress and ultimately, coaching burnout. Successful coaches are altruistic leaders who place the needs of their athletes above their own, and often above those of their partners, spouses, and families. It has been said that coaches raise everyone else's children but their own. For this reason, one of the most often-cited reasons for over-dedicated coaches who retire prematurely from the coaching profession is "to spend more time with their families."

Self-care skills that coaches promote for their athletes, namely, nutrition, exercise, rest, and restoration, and environment are often neglected for themselves and result in the inability of the coach to lead a balanced and healthy lifestyle. For this reason, sports psychology professionals encourage coaches to take care of themselves by integrating a variety of recreational (daily exercise, hobbies, vacations, etc.), educational (time management techniques, relaxation strategies, etc.) work-related (delegate authority and responsibly, change jobs, change positions [become an assistant coach if head coaching is overwhelming]), and social strategies (seek social support, associated with or make friends who are not coworkers, etc.) that will prevent and reverse coaching burnout.

HOLISTIC COACHING

The world of the coach is multifaceted and diverse, but one leadership concept is at the core of effective coaching; the athlete meets sport at the coach. The coach is the definer, creator, provider, and deliverer of the sport experience to the athlete. The sport experience is necessarily a direct reflection of the coach, and of the coach's philosophy, beliefs, values, principles, and priorities. The quality of an athlete's experience can never exceed the quality of the leadership providing it.

As stated previously, the statement "coach the person first, and the sport second" is sound advice for coaches at all levels. A holistic approach to coaching can go a long way in helping coaches to be effective educators and leaders in a contemporary world of the millennium athlete. Such a world is oftentimes characterized by "forced achievement" and rising expectations. Young persons today are constantly "playing up" in the current age of specialization; an impatient age that ignores developmental readiness. Immersion in such a world, without proper leadership and perspective, can result in not only the loss of one's performance effectiveness, but also the loss of one's love and passion for sport.

A holistic coaching and leadership style is directed toward meeting the needs of athletic participants by providing both on- and off-the-field educational opportunities for self-improvement. In this approach to coaching, athletic participation and performance are viewed in the context of one's lifestyle and provides athletes with the academic/educational, life, and athletic skill sets to succeed in sport and life.

Mastery of life, academic, and athletic skill sets can help athletes of all developmental levels respond effectively to the demands of an athletic lifestyle. Ensuring success both on and off the athletic field is dependent on an athlete's ability to lead a healthy lifestyle in pursuit of athletic excellence. By providing essential resources for growth, academic and athletic skill development will go a long way toward building success-ful athletic programs, in part based on attracting and retaining happy, healthy, confident, and effective team members.

Life Skills

It is often the case that just as we are about to do great things, life gets in the way. This is certainly true for athletes who do not possess the life skills to prevent the negative spillover of stress into their on-the-field performances. Due to an increasing emphasis on academic perfor-mance during the high school years, for example, the acquisition of life skills has been put on the back burner for many young student-athletes. Life skills include but are not limited to time management, decision making, nutrition, assertiveness training, anger management, human sexuality, self-care through relaxation and sleep, financial management, and social, communication, and leadership skills.

It is often taken for granted that these skills are learned either at home or in school. The reality is that many athletes are not mastering life skills at every educational level. Integrating life skills training into existing athletic programs can help coaches and athletes identify re-sources in time of need. Most importantly, integrating these services into an athletic program can prevent the occurrence of lifestyle-driven performance blocks and decrements.

Academic Skills

Academic advising is an essential part of the formula for a successful experience at all educational levels. Academic skills include under-standing academic workloads and course requirements, learning how and what to study, mastering time management, seeking academic help from teachers, acquiring test-taking skills and strategies, developing research and writing skills, juggling in-season travel and academic responsibilities, learning to use library resources, and getting the most out of existing academic support services and programs.

Coaches are teachers, and as teachers, they must build or provide resources that will help develop a student-athlete's academic and athletic confidence. Identifying academically at-risk student-athletes is essential to retaining student-athletes in educational athletic programs.

Most student-athletes are at risk because of the physical demands of their sport. Many are capable of earning good grades, but are simply too tired to pursue academic excellence. Proper rest, recovery, nutrition, and sleep are essential for sound academic and athletic performance. Blending academic, training, travel, and competition schedules requires careful and flexible planning, especially for at risk student-athletes.

Athletic Skills

In addition to mastering the physical skills necessary for success in any sport, athletes can also improve their performance effectiveness by mastering the mental skill sets that can affect performance outcomes. Developing a mental game to compliment an athlete's physical skills enables athletes to mentally and physically prepare themselves for the performance challenges they may face in competitive athletic settings.

Athletic-oriented mental skills include but are not limited to: avoiding overtraining, responding to and coping with athletic injury, visualization and mental rehearsal, concentration skills, communication skills with coaches, positive self-talk, constructive performance evaluation, goal setting and attainment strategies and techniques, understanding and thriving on athletic motivation, composure skills, mental preparation strategies for practice and performance settings, and preparing for life after sport.

Contemporary coaches realize that it is necessary to provide the support services and personnel necessary to complement the goals of the athletes they coach. In addition to the coaching staff, coaches can provide personnel and educational programs available to team members by incorporating sports psychology professionals, counselors, and academic advisors to present programs and work with athletes on an individual basis as needed.

Sports psychology professionals can also enhance athletic performance by providing mental skills training in concentration, confidence, composure, and commitment. After working so hard to recruit and develop your team members, finding professionals to deliver these services is an important insurance policy.

PUTTING IT ALL TOGETHER

In the final analysis, coaches are influential educators who have the opportunity to promote personal excellence through athletic participation. Self-care, self-responsibility, self-improvement, and self-forgiveness are the pillars of personal excellence in sport and life. These attributes can be effectively cultivated and taught by coaches who possess a sound understanding of the psychosocial aspects of coaching and leadership.

RECOMMENDED READING

Janssen, J. (1999). *Championship team building: What every coach needs to know to build a motivated, committed and cohesive team*. Tucson, AZ: Winning the Mental Game.

Janssen, J., & Dale, G. (2002). *The seven secrets of successful coaches: How to unlock and unleash your team's full potential*. Tucson, AZ: Winning the Mental Game.

McGuire, R. (2005). Winning kids with sport: A construction model for positive coaching. In R. A. Vernacchia & T. A. Statler (Eds.), *The psychology of high-performance track and field* (pp. 28–34). Mountain View, CA: Track & Field News.

Vernacchia, R. A. (2003). *Inner strength: The mental dynamics of athletic performance*. Palo Alto, CA: Warde.

Vernacchia, R. A., McGuire, R. T., & Cook, D. L. (1996). *Coaching mental excellence: "It does matter whether you win or lose . . . "* Portola Valley, CA: Warde.

Chapter 4

A Psychological Approach toward Understanding and Preventing the Overtraining Syndrome

John S. Raglin and Göran Kenttä

Athletes use every resource available in the effort to push themselves to ever higher levels of performance. These improvements are the consequence of factors ranging from innovative equipment to the application of research findings from sport science disciplines such as nutrition, hydration, and biomechanics. Advances in the treatment and rehabilitation of injury have also allowed athletes to continue participating at high levels with injuries that in the past would have been career-ending. Taking these and other contributing factors into consideration though, experts generally regard the most important factor to be changes in the way athletes train, specifically the increase in training loads. In many cases the evolution of training practices has been dramatic. In 1954, Roger Bannister was the first human to run a sub-four-minute mile. He achieved this feat while a full-time medical student and was limited to no more than 30 minutes of training a day (2004), a duration that many contemporary athletes would spend merely warming up. Mark Spitz swam his way to Olympic gold medals in world-record times at the Munich Olympics in 1972 by training a maximum distance of 10,000 yards a day, a volume that many age-group swimmers matched or even exceeded within two decades. This trend toward greater training has also become evident in team sports, racket sports, and non-endurance events where there is a growing premium to achieve peak athletic conditioning.

Along with the rise in training loads, it has become common to train and compete year-round in many sports, even for young athletes. This raises the question as to how long these practices can continue before records stop falling or athletes begin to break down. In fact, it has been long recognized that training regimens that improve performance for the majority of athletes will paradoxically have dire consequences for other individuals of equal skill and conditioning, a phenomenon described in the medical literature over a hundred years ago. This condition was initially referred to as staleness or the staleness syndrome, but currently it is more generally called the overtraining syndrome (OTS). Other, less frequently used labels include the unexplained underperformance syndrome (UPS), inadequate recovery syndrome (IRS), and non-functional overreaching (NFOR). The defining symptom of OTS is a serious loss in the capacity to train and compete at customary levels that persists for several weeks or longer. Importantly, this performance decrement is deemed to be precipitated by training stress paired with insufficient recovery rather than from a preexisting condition such as an illness or injury. Other factors, particularly psychosocial stressors, are regarded to be secondary contributors to the condition, but research quantifying their influence is lacking. The initial stage of OTS, or cases in which performance has stagnated or is just beginning to deteriorate, is referred to as overreaching, and can usually be treated with short periods of reduced training or with a short layoff of a few days. There is some debate as to the role of overreaching as some researchers regard it as an undesirable condition that should always be avoided, whereas others consider it is a useful or even necessary phase in a training regimen that, if carefully managed, will result in a greater training adaptation and improvements in athletic performance. Aside from the chronic loss of performance, OTS is associated with a large number of signs and symptoms that occur with varying frequency. Among the most common are medical illnesses such as upper-respiratory infections and mood disturbances, particularly depression. Various behavioral symptoms have been noted, including sleep disturbances (longer sleep onset, frequent awakening, poor sleep quality) and a loss of appetite. Perceptual changes are also common, including increased perception of effort for training and competition, muscle soreness, and feelings of heaviness in the arms and legs.

There is evidence that some athletes who experience OTS may be at an increased risk of developing burnout, which in turn may precipitate a withdrawal from the sport entirely. Burnout has been defined as a persistent condition associated with work settings that is "primarily characterized by exhaustion, which is accompanied by distress, a sense of reduced effectiveness, decreased motivation, and the development of dysfunctional attitude and behaviors at work" (Schaufeli & Enzmann, 1998, p. 36). It is important to emphasize that the original literature on burnout addresses very different samples and precipitating conditions than overtraining, yet sports psychologists have often regarded these conditions as synonymous. Moreover, only limited empirical research has been published on burnout with athletes, and the extant literature indicates that they are distinct conditions that require different treatment interventions. The primary distinction noted in the literature is that many athletes with OTS still report being motivated to continue training and competing whereas athletes suffering from burnout exhibit a loss of motivation and are contemplating quitting or retiring from their sport.

TREATMENT

In the earliest descriptions of overtraining, the need for rest was recognized; athletes have been advised to stop training in their sport for a period of weeks if not longer. Rest does not mean complete inactivity, and athletes should be encouraged to participate in recreational activities or other moderately vigorous pursuits that they enjoy. Medical testing is recommended, not only to rule out other conditions and illnesses that share similar symptoms with OTS, but also to initiate treatment for colds and other infectious disorders common in athletes with OTS. Because it has been found that upwards of 80 percent of athletes with OTS exhibit depression of clinical severity, psychological treatment has also been recommended. This may involve counseling or other forms of cognitive therapy, but in more severe cases, medication may be necessary. There is no evidence that standard sports-psychology performance interventions (e.g., imagery, goal setting) are beneficial.

PREVALENCE

While OTS has been regarded to be a problem endemic to athletes who train intensively for most any sport, there has been little published information as to its prevalence. Survey research involving collegiate swimmers and other endurance athletes undergoing competitive training have reported the yearly rate of OTS to average approximately 10 percent (range: 7–21%) but the higher percentages reported in some studies may be inflated because of merging cases of both overtrained and overreached athletes. In the first investigation on the lifetime prevalence of OTS, it was found that fully 60 percent of elite female and 64 percent of elite male distance runners reported experiencing one or more episode of OTS during their running careers, whereas the rate dropped to 33 percent for nonelite adult runners. Notably, the weekly training mileage of these runners was significantly lower than the elite athletes, supporting the view that the exposure to training directly increases the risk of OTS, regardless of athlete status (i.e., elite or nonelite). These results also indicate that male and female athletes who undergo comparable training loads are at similar risk of OTS, whereas earlier reports suggested that females were less likely to be affected.

More recent reports indicate the rate of OTS in young athletes to be comparable with findings for adults. In a study involving 231 age-group swimmers from four countries, Raglin et al. (2000) had participants complete a questionnaire in which they were queried about their training practices and whether they had ever become over-trained. It was found that 34.6 percent of the entire sample reported at least one case of overtraining (R: 20.5% to 45.1%), which persisted for an average of 3.6 weeks. These athletes had faster personal best times in the 100-meter freestyle and were involved in the sport for a longer period of time than swimmers who had never had a case of OTS (6.0 versus 4.9 years), consistent with the findings involving adult runners.

Athletes who have developed OTS appear to be at a greater risk of developing it again. Among freshmen varsity swimmers who developed OTS during their first collegiate training season of training, 91 percent became overtrained again one or more times during the following three years of training, whereas the rate was only 34 percent in swimmers who did not develop OTS their freshman year. A higher-than-expected rate of OTS has also been found in elite Swedish junior skiers who became overtrained during their first competitive high school season. Whether these findings indicate some individuals are inherently prone to developing OTS when exposed to overload training, or whether succumbing to OTS raises the risk of relapse, is yet unclear, but both possibilities reinforce the importance of preventing athletes from ever developing the disorder.

PREVENTION STRATEGIES

It is clearly preferable to prevent athletes from becoming overtrained than having to treat them. Although most experts would agree that OTS can be avoided by not training intensively, this is not a sensible option for either the aspiring athlete or coach. Consequently, attention has turned to identifying symptoms or markers that can be used to reliably diagnose athletes in the early stages of OTS where short-term reductions in training or rest periods are likely to be effective. Most of this research has focused on traditional exercise physiology measures involving cardiovascular, metabolic, and hormonal variables. The timing or setting of these tests has utilized resting conditions as well as both during and following recovery from standardized exercise or sport tests of strength or endurance.

The first major review of this literature was published over two decades ago (Kuipers & Keizer, 1988), and the authors concluded that useful markers of OTS had yet not yet been identified. A follow-up review by Fry and associates (1991) identified over 80 potential markers of OTS that had been examined in the published literature, yet concluded that: "At present there is no one single diagnostic test that can define overtraining" (p. 32). Despite considerable research in the years since these initial reviews, the goal of identifying a reliable marker of OTS remains elusive. In perhaps the most comprehensive recent review of the literature published to date, Urhausen and Kindermann (2002) concluded that "there has been little improvement in recent years in the tools available for the diagnosis of OTS" (p. 95).

Despite these disappointing findings, literature reviews have identified a number of physiological variables that do reliably change in accordance with training volume or intensity but fail to distinguish between healthy (i.e., adaptive responses to training) and overtrained athletes (i.e., maladaptive responses to training). A smaller subset of physiological markers have been found to exhibit at least some degree of specificity for identifying OTS, and these include reduced muscle glycogen, elevated cortisol, and decreased leptin. However, for a marker to be of practical value, it must respond during the initial phase when an athlete is overreached rather than overtrained. If it changes only after the athlete has a fully developed case of OTS, then it is of little value beyond corroborating a diagnosis. Because performance decrements indicative of overreaching or OTS can begin to occur following intensive training programs as brief as a few days in duration, a useful diagnostic measure should be able to be taken daily and provide results with little or no delay. These requirements rule out physiological markers that involve technically demanding procedures or time-consuming analytical procedures (e.g., cortisol). Another serious limitation is that many physiological markers require invasive procedures (e.g., blood drawing or muscle biopsy).

Because of the previously described concerns along with the fact that most physiological measures are not useful in identifying OTS, researchers have turned to examining other categories of markers of staleness, particularly self-report measures including assessments of mood and motivation, perception (ratings of perceived exertion, soreness, fatigue, heaviness), and behaviors (sleep, appetite). Among these variables there is evidence that validated psychological measures, particularly mood states, are more consistently associated with training load and OTS compared to the majority of biological measures. In addition, self-reports are also advantageous because they can be completed and scored quickly in the field at little cost. However, it is crucial that psychological measures be administered and interpreted by individuals with appropriate training. In order to reduce the occurrence of response distortion, whereby psychological questionnaires are completed in a uniformly positive manner regardless of how individuals actually feel, it is important to ensure the confidentiality of study participants. Another option is to have study participants also complete so-called "lie scales," which can detect cases of response distortion, but this procedure has only rarely been used in overtraining research.

MOOD STATE MONITORING DURING SPORT TRAINING

The potential efficacy of psychological monitoring was first recognized by William Morgan and colleagues at the University of Wisconsin, who initiated a long-term study of the mood state response of college swimmers during their training season. Their research utilized the Profile of Mood States, or POMS (McNair, Lorr, & Dropplemann, 1992), a 65-item Likert format questionnaire that measures the psychological factors of tension, depression, anger, vigor, fatigue, and confusion. Morgan combined these mood variables to create a more general, global measure of mood disturbance by summing the negative POMS factors (Tension, Depression, Anger, Fatigue, Confusion), subtracting the positive POMS factor of Vigor and adding a constant of 100. This measure has since been adopted by the developers of the POMS and has been widely used in studies of both athletes and nonathletes. Based on the standard instructions, individuals respond to each POMS item according to how they have been feeling "last week including today." This results in moderately stable mood measures (r_{tt} = .45 – .74) that are unaffected by a single treatment or stressors of brief duration, but which can be altered by persisting stimuli such as chronic sport training.

Initial research revealed that periods of intensive training resulted in significant increases in the negative POMS factors and a decrease in vigor in swimmers who at the outset of the season exhibited positive scores on all the POMS factors, widely referred to as the iceberg profile and commonly found in successful athletes across many sports. This finding led to follow-up studies in which the POMS was administered more frequently during training on a monthly or even weekly basis. The results of this work indicated that each increase in training load was closely tied to a corresponding elevation in mood disturbance, with the most severe mood disturbances occurring during peak training. Decreases in or tapering of training loads resulted in improvements in mood state, and by the end of the training season, mood state scores had returned to their preseason values for most of the athletes. This dose-response relationship between training load and mood state did not differ in the men and women swimmers except in cases in which the teams underwent significantly different training regimens. Figure 4.1 presents a typical example for a college swimming team. Subsequent research by Morgan and other researchers

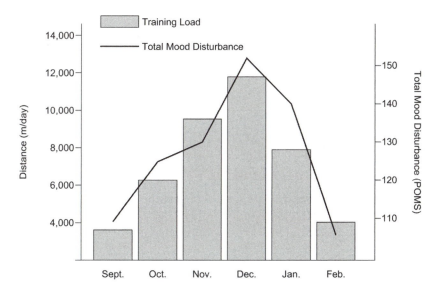

Figure 4.1. Changes in POMS total mood disturbance scores during a training season in a sample of college varsity swimmers.

has replicated these findings in other athletes in a variety of endurance sports as well as non-endurance sports that incorporate rigorous training regimens.

Similar dose-response relationships have been observed using other self-report Likert-scales of mood and other variables including perception of effort, muscle soreness, and feelings of heaviness, although the degree to which these factors change in response to heavy training differs. In a study of age-group young swimmers from four countries (Raglin et al., 2000), a consistent trend was found for self-reports of feelings of heaviness to increase the most during hard training, followed by perceived exertion of training, whereas sleep and appetite were the least altered (Figure 4.2).

The majority of POMS overtraining studies have involved assessments throughout an entire competitive season (i.e., 4 to 6 months) but for some sports it is common to have training camps or programs in which large increases in training are rapidly implemented during a period that may be as brief as a few days. In this case the instructions of the POMS are altered, with athletes responding according to how they are feeling "today" or "right now," yielding a *state* measure of

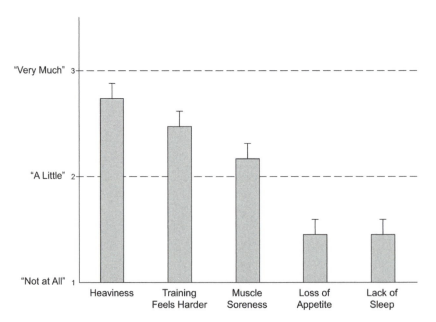

Figure 4.2. Mean ratings of training-related perceptions of young swimmers during peak training. (Adapted from Raglin et al. [2000], *Pediatric sport science*)

mood responsive to acute stressors and that can change in intensity across a brief period of time (e.g., hours or minutes). The results of this research reveal that little as 2 to 4 days of intensified training (> of 50% baseline training) can result in significant increases mood disturbances (Raglin & Wilson, 2000). In research that included physiological measures, cortisol and heart rate remained unchanged, indicating that psychological assessments are more responsive to the acute stressors imposed by rapid elevations in training.

MOOD DISTURBANCES IN HEALTHY AND OVERTRAINED ATHLETES

Although the finding that mood state is consistently altered by changes in training load is notable, the more important practical concern is whether mood differs between athletes who successfully adapt to hard training and those who develop OTS. This research paradigm has involved either contrasting mood state values during a training season between team members identified by their coaches as overreached or overtrained with those who underwent the same training regiment but who remained free of the disorder, or subjecting research participants to standardized training protocols and comparing the responses of those who adapt with athletes who are experiencing signs of overreaching. In the latter case it should be emphasized that when individuals showed signs of overreaching, the training was terminated as it would be unethical to intentionally produce OTS. The results of this work indicate that during periods of intensive training, total mood disturbance scores are consistently higher in athletes showing signs of overreaching or OTS, although exceptions have been noted.

There is also evidence that pattern of mood-specific disturbances is unique in overtrained athletes, an observation that provides further support for the potential of the POMS as a practical tool. Studies of collegiate swimmers indicate the POMS factors of fatigue and vigor exhibit the largest shifts from easy to peak training among athletes who remain free from OTS, with depression exhibiting the smallest elevation among the remaining POMS factors. Athletes with OTS exhibited a different pattern; in addition to larger shifts in all the POMS factors, it was found that depression exhibited the largest elevation of any single POMS factor. Other research involving overtrained swimmers has found that POMS depression scores were significantly correlated with salivary cortisol, implicating the involvement of a central dysregulation in the Hypothalamic-Pituitary-Adrenal axis.

ENHANCING THE POMS TO ASSESS OVERTRAINING RESPONSES

Although the previously described research indicates the POMS has potential in identifying individuals at risk of developing OTS, several factors may constrain its efficacy in identifying overtrained athletes. Aside from the potential occurrence of response distortion, the POMS subscales vary in their sensitivity to the stress of athletic training. Some factors, particularly confusion, have been found to be relatively insensitive even to intense overload training. Other work indicates that some POMS factors are sensitive to stressors unrelated to OTS. Unlike other POMS factors, scores on the tension variable often remain elevated or even increase during training tapers in college swimmers, and it has been speculated that this reflects the impending stress of major competition.

More fundamentally, the POMS was designed for general use and not specifically for athlete samples or sport settings. In the field of sports psychology, there is a long-standing practice to employ sport-specific psychological measures under the belief that existing measures are insensitive or too general to assess to the unique environment of sports or characteristics of athletes. Therefore, researchers have developed over 300 sport-specific psychological measures of personality, motivation, and mood to be used in specific sport situations (e.g., competition) or groups (e.g., runners). Unfortunately, many of these scales have not been adequately validated, and so their efficacy remains to be demonstrated.

In an effort to enhance the sensitivity of the POMS to detect OTS, Raglin and Morgan (1994) analyzed mood responses in a sample of 186 college varsity swimmers who had undergone mood testing throughout their training. Statistical procedures were used to identify the POMS items that responded to the greatest degree among those athletes who were showing signs of overtraining (i.e., overreaching) or were diagnosed with OTS. The analyses identified five items from the POMS depression scale and two from the anger scale. This seven-item pool was labeled the Training Distress Scale (TDS) and subjected to additional testing. A subsequent analysis examined whether the TDS would be more accurate in identifying athletes with OTS compared to the standard POMS subscales using a sample of 29 college track-and-field athletes who completed the POMS during their most intense phase of training. The team coach identified six athletes in the sample who were experiencing performance problems directly attributable to overreaching or OTS. The researchers anticipated that athletes who possessed mood disturbance scores one or more standard deviations above the mean value for the entire team would be either overreached or overtrained, and assignments using the TDS were compared to those made based on the POMS total mood disturbance score as well as the POMS depression scale in order to compare their relative efficacy. It was found that predictions using each of the POMS scales correctly identified overreached and overtrained athletes at rates that exceeded chance ($P < .05$), but the TDS was more specific and resulted in fewer false positives (i.e., predicting OTS when athletes were actually healthy) compared with those based on either total mood disturbance or depression scores. The TDS has since been translated into several languages and found to be efficacious in assessing mood changes during age-group athletes. Specifically, TDS scores were higher in young athletes who reported symptoms of staleness compared with healthy competitors.

Other scales have been developed by researchers who contend that measures specifically devised to assess overtraining and recovery should provide even greater efficacy than general psychological measures such as the POMS. Unlike the TDS, which was established using empirical procedures, these scales were created according to theoretical assumptions about what psychological and behavior factors should be associated with OTS. The most extensively studied instrument has been the RESTQ (Kellman & Kallus, 2001), a 76-item questionnaire encompassing 19 separate factors that assess both overtraining and recovery responses in endurance athletes. Initial work indicates that the RESTQ can identify athletes with signs of staleness, but accuracy rates have not been published, nor has the efficacy of this measure been directly compared to the POMS or other scales.

Some research has been conducted to determine if mood state monitoring can be used as a practical means to reduce the occurrence of OTS in athletes who must undergo intensive overload training. In the most ambitious of these studies, Berglund and Safstrom (1994) used the Swedish language version of the POMS to conduct weekly assessments in elite men and women race canoeists who were training for the Olympics. Using each athlete's own baseline total mood disturbance score as a criterion, when an athlete's own total mood disturbance score exceeded baseline by at least 50 percent, training was reduced until scores fell to within 10 percent of the baseline. In contrast, low mood disturbance scores were regarded by the authors as indicative of undertraining. Consequently, such cases lead to increasing training loads until mood disturbance scores rose to a point regarded as indicative of beneficial overreaching. Of the entire sample, 64 percent had training reduced at some point and 57 percent had training increased, indicating that some athletes required each intervention during different phases of the training program. None of the athletes developed signs of OTS, a decrease in the average 10 percent rate found in previous training seasons. Although these results are promising, further testing of this and similar approaches is needed involving larger samples and non-intervention control conditions. If these results are replicable and generalize to other sports, then mood state monitoring in combination with selected physiological assessments, may well provide an effective means of reducing the risk of OTS in competitive athletes while also potentiating the performance benefiting effects of intense training.

GENERAL SUMMARY

Intensive physical conditioning is a necessary aspect for most sports, yet it is inherently stressful and results in both physiological and psychological disturbances. Fortunately, most athletes are able not only to tolerate this stress, but to adapt to it with improved performances. For reasons that remain poorly understood, some athletes fail to adapt and develop the overtraining syndrome, suffering from chronic performance decrements that persist for weeks or months. While physiological research on OTS has enhanced our understanding of the disorder, the findings of this work have had little practical impact for coaches and athletes; OTS remains an intractable problem that has resisted the concerted efforts of scientists, coaches, and trainers to prevent it. However, a growing body of research indicates that mood state and other psychological variables are closely associated with training volume, both with schedules that are altered gradually across a period of weeks or months and those that are more rapidly altered. Furthermore, both the magnitude of disturbance and specific pattern of mood disturbance is unique in athletes with OTS, and some research has exploited these findings to successfully prevent the occurrence of OTS by altering training loads in response to mood changes. Several recently developed questionnaires have been created specifically to assess the psychological consequences of OTS, but even if research proves these scales to provide enhanced sensitivity and specificity over extant measures, their efficacy will be further enhanced by integrating mood assessments into a more comprehensive monitoring strategy integrating relevant physiological, performance, and nutritional information.

The approach of using mood state monitoring to examine the issue of overtraining is a telling example of how carefully conducted sports psychology research can contribute to our understanding of difficult problems in sports and exercise. The complexity of the overtraining syndrome compellingly demonstrates that most phenomena in sports are best understood as psychobiological rather than either physiological or psychological. Moreover, it is an example in which the experience of stress, if managed appropriately, is ultimately beneficial. This perspective has recently become accepted, if not embraced by exercise scientists but was recognized long ago by the father of American sports psychology, Coleman Roberts Griffith, who stated: "The athlete, at work and at play constitutes a fine laboratory for the study of vexing physiological and psychological problems, many of which are distorted by the attempt to reduce them to simpler terms" (Griffith, 1929, p. vii). Researchers and coaches would be wise to follow his advice.

RECOMMENDED READING

Morgan, W. P., Brown, D. R., Raglin, J. S., O'Connor, P. J., & Ellickson, K. A. (1987). Psychological monitoring of overtraining and staleness. *British Journal of Sports Medicine, 21*, 107–114.

Raglin, J. S. (1993). Overtraining and staleness: Psychometric monitoring of endurance athletes. In: R. N. Singer, M. Murphey, & L. K. Tennant (Eds.), *Handbook of Research on Sport Psychology.* (pp. 840–850). New York: Macmillan.

Urhausen, A. & Kindermann, W. (2002). Diagnosis of overtraining: What tools do we have? *Sports Medicine, 32*, 95–102.

REFERENCES

Bannister, R. (2004). *The Four-minute mile.* Guilford, CT: The Lyons Press.

Berglund, B., & Säfström, H. (1994). Psychological monitoring and modulation of training load of world-class canoeists. *Medicine and Science in Sports and Exercise, 26*, 1036–1040.

Fry, R. W., Morton, A. R., & Keast, D. (1991). Overtraining in athletes: An update. *Sports Medicine, 12*, 32–65.

Griffith, C. R. (1929). *The psychology of coaching.* New York: Charles Scribner's Sons.

Kellmann, M. & Kallus, K. W. (2001). Recovery stress questionnaire for athletes: User manual. Champaign, IL: Human Kinetics.

Kuipers, H., & Keizer, H. A. (1988). Overtraining in elite athletes: Review and directions for the future. *Sports Medicine, 6*, 248–252.

McNair, D. M., Lorr, M., & Droppleman, L. F. (1992). *Manual for the profile of mood states*. San Diego, CA: Educational and Industrial Testing Service.

Raglin, J. S., & Wilson, G. (2000). Overtraining and staleness in athletes. In: Y. L. Hanin (Ed.), *Emotions in sports* (pp. 191–207). Champaign, IL: Human Kinetics.

Raglin, J. S., Sawamura, S., Alexiou, S., Hassmén, P., & Kenttä, G. (2000). Training practices and staleness in 13–18 year old swimmers: A cross-cultural study. *Pediatric Sports Medicine, 12,* 61–70.

Schaufeli, W., & Enzmann, D. (1998). *The burnout companion to study and practice: A critical analysis*. Philadelphia: Taylor & Francis.

Urhausen, A. & Kindermann, W. (2002). Diagnosis of overtraining: What tools do we have? *Sports Medicine, 32,* 95–102.

Yerkes, R. M., & Dodson, J. D. (1908). The relation of strength of stimulus to rapidity of habit formation. *Journal of Comparative Neurology of Psychology,* 18, 459–482.

Chapter 5

Personality: Contributions to Performance, Injury Risk, and Rehabilitation

Frank M. Webbe, Christine M. Salinas, Stephanie J. Tiedemann, and Kristy Quackenbush

To the casual onlooker, it might appear that knowledge and study of the role of personality factors in sport would be a gold mine of information. Indeed, a search of the twentieth-century literature in sports psychology that focused on personality produces a large output, testimony to this interest. It seems intuitive that that the core traits and tendencies that define a person should be critical predictors of success, reliability, socialization on a team, performance, and ultimately, winning. Moreover, one could easily accept that narrow personality profiles might predispose for more or less success in specific sports. For example, the notion that an internal focus and a certain degree of independence should predict better adaptation in individual sports such as golf or tennis appears almost obvious.

The casual onlooker would be surprised to find that what appears to be both credible and obvious has only limited empirical support within the literature of sport psychology. In this chapter we summarize much that is known about the relationship between personality variables and sport-related performance and behavior. We review briefly the constructs of personality that inform sports psychology research. We cover in depth the person-oriented factors that define risk of athletic injury as well as recovery from injury, perhaps the soundest personality models in sports psychology.

PERSONALITY IN THE HISTORY OF SPORTS PSYCHOLOGY

Personality is a construct, a convenient invention used to summarize individual tendencies, attitudes, and behaviors. Some years ago, Rainer Martens (1975) created a graphic description of personality in the form of a pyramid, with the base containing the psychological core of the person, the middle area containing typical or default responses, and the upper tip containing the socially governed role-related behaviors (see Figure 5.1). Martens's approach at once repudiated the notion that enduring traits were critical variables in explaining the variability in sports performance and established the necessity for more extensive modeling of variables critical for understanding and prediction.

Martens argued that native traits as causes for behavior were insufficient to explain the variability in performance both within and between individuals. Typical responses could be seen as representing both dispositional traits and learned responses, whereas role-related behaviors encompass clearly learned, often socially structured behaviors. Trait, situational, and phenomenological approaches have all received support

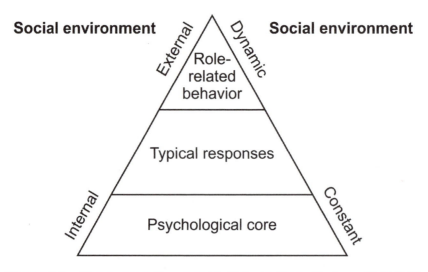

Figure 5.1. The personality pyramid. (Adapted from Martens, R. [1975]. *Social psychology and physical activity.* New York: Harper & Row)

as useful concepts for explaining sport-related behavior. However, the interactional approach that combines these three constructs remains as the primary personality model in modern sports psychology. Traits are seen as highly individual and likely reflective of genetic influences and are relatively stable over time. Although the potential utility of a psychodynamic approach in explaining how early childhood experiences might mold core tendencies sounds promising, the difficulty of empirical investigation has stunted any real influence in modern personality studies in sports psychology. Nonetheless, the basic question as to whether individuals are born with innate traits that govern behavior, or whether early childhood experiences mold such traits remains elusive. Such nature-nurture questions are both the bane of psychology and, at the same time, the spice that makes things interesting. The newer phenomenological perspective has added a very attractive psychological topping to Marten's original pyramid. According to this approach, one's experience of events as well as how those events make one feel is seen as exerting powerful influence over the actual effects of such events. For example, Selye's original theory of stress suggested that all stress has deleterious effects on the body. The phenomenological approach suggests that only those events viewed as negative will cause harmful stress. The positive stress that might arise from feelings of love or anticipation of competition might not degrade bodily functions in the same manner.

In sports psychology, trait approaches have been used extensively to identify enduring qualities and characteristics of individuals that relate to success and failure within the sport context. For example, tough-mindedness is a construct often employed to explain why some athletes endure and overcome obstacles while others give in and give up. Is tough-mindedness something that a person is born with, or is it something that is learned through a reinforcement and punishment history inculcated by the family and extended environment, beginning in childhood? Obviously, it may be either. The usual experimental controls that are employed to tease out nature versus nurture—such as twin studies—are infrequently applied in sport. Therefore, although the origin of traits that seem predictive of performance, success, and failure, may not be available to us, the impact may still stand out clearly. The causal relationship of traits to sport performance also may be cloudy, since rarely are true experiments possible when dealing with human participants. This, of course, does not stop proponents of specific theories from asserting causal influences in either direction. For example, the great baseball promoter (and former big league pitcher) Albert Goodwill Spalding once asserted that "the average boy who loves baseball is not the sort of boy who loves to go off with a gun intent on killing some poor bird. Baseball has done a lot to keep the Yankee lad from being brutal." Historically, investigation of the role of personality variables in sports psychology was secondary to social factors, but just barely. Triplett's 1895 report of social factors that facilitated the performance of cyclists is generally credited as the origin of modern sports psychology. That empirical report was followed just four years later by Scripture's case-study/anecdotal account of the role of personality factors in shaping the character of sports participants. Thankfully, Scripture was more scientific in his pronouncements than Mr. Spalding.

PERSONALITY AND ATHLETIC PERFORMANCE

A common anecdote that many coaches use in sports when encouraging their athletes is that "sports is 20% physical and 80% mental," a welcome variant from Yogi Berra's observation that "sport is 90% mental and the other half physical." As described earlier, personality is a set of enduring characteristics that differentiate people and are typically exhibited in one's behaviors, thoughts, and emotions. Within the sports context, competitiveness, aggression, the will to win, leadership ability, mental toughness, and other features of personality may determine athletic success. This section summarizes how various personal characteristics may be at work in the athletic arena.

Although no athletic personality profile has withstood the test of time, there are common personality traits and levels of traits that seem to differentiate athletes from nonathletes. For example, athletes tend to be more extroverted, self-confident, competitive, and dominant than nonathletes. Moreover, certain qualities, such as an athlete's ability to cope with stress and the way in which he or she perceives stress, likely affect their ability to succeed in the sports realm. Other evidence suggests that athletes who can more easily get "into the zone" and experience "flow," a time when an athlete is fully engaged in the activity that he or she is performing so that it feels effortless, may predict athletic success. Tiger Woods and LeBron James are prime examples of athletes who embody these characteristics even in the most stressful athletic circumstances. Personality traits may also influence the manner in which an athlete trains for competition or reacts to a coach's feedback, both of which influence athletic performance. For example, those who are highly conscientious and open to new experiences may practice more often; may be more diligent in targeting areas of weakness; and may more readily accept constructive criticism of their game. Other evidence shows that personality flaws may be associated with reduced athletic performance. Within youth sports, boys with Attention Deficit Hyperactivity Disorder (ADHD) exhibit higher levels of aggression and subsequent disqualification across several sports than boys without ADHD. In adults, athletes who view their stress as a threat tend to have less team loyalty, which has been shown to have a negative impact on performance.

Self-efficacy, or one's belief of being capable, can contribute to an athlete's level of performance. For example, athletes who believe strongly in themselves will likely outperform their equally skilled counterparts who exhibit self-doubt. In this way, an athlete's positive perception appears to be linked to real success on the court or field. Thus, the battle between rivals may be won well before the game clock has even been turned on.

Sensation seeking, or the seeking of new, varied, or intense experiences, can also help or hinder a player's performance. When a soccer player takes a risk by successfully attempting a goal from a far distance or a quarterback is willing to try a new play spontaneously on a 3rd down to gain extra yardage, high levels of the trait we call sensation seeking may bolster the athlete's inherent talent. However, sensation seeking can also be an athlete's adversary. This is apparent when a basketball player takes a jump shot impulsively and misses, giving the other team possession at the end of the game; or when a defensive player goes for a steal at an inopportune time and instead gets a foul called, resulting in the other team gaining additional points. The line between success and failure is a fine one. Although Michael Jordan may have been the most successful basketball player ever in making winning shots with seconds remaining in a game, he also missed many buzzer beaters. Yet like the grin of the Cheshire Cat in *Alice in Wonderland*, the made shots remain vivid in our memories, and the missed shots have faded. The critical factor with Jordan and others was the confidence and self-belief, not the failure.

Perhaps the most famous statement of and graphic portrayal of the relationship of mood state to performance was the so-called "iceberg profile" described by Morgan (1979) to differentiate elite from nonelite athletes. Using the Profile of Mood States with its six subscales, Morgan described a profile wherein successful athletes showed a peak on the vigor subscales, and decreasing levels on the various negative mood scales (tension, confusion, depression, fatigue, and anger). As shown

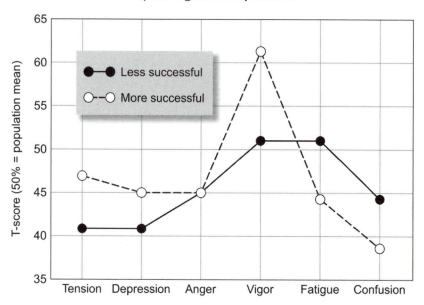

Figure 5.2. The Iceberg profile. (Adapted from Morgan, W. [1979]. Prediction of performance in athletics. In P. Klavora and J. W. Daniel, eds., *Coach, athlete and the sport psychologist.* Champaign, IL: Human Kinetics)

in Figure 5.2, in comparison to the successful athletes, less successful athletes had a flatter profile (or one with peaks on one or more of the negative mood subscales).

Although Morgan and other authors collected data in support of the iceberg profile as predictive of athletic success, a very comprehensive meta-analysis of 33 studies that used the Profile of Mood States (POMS) and reported some measure of performance outcome showed that actual differences in profiles were extremely small. The authors rightly cautioned against using this or any other single measure to understand or predict athletic success.

Motivation

Ray and Wiese-Bjornstal (1999) describe motivation as a "state of readiness or eagerness to pursue an action or to change." An athlete's motivation can affect the desire to train, which can in turn affect the ability to compete effectively. There are intrinsic and extrinsic motivators for athletes, both of which can enhance athletic performance by encouraging an athlete to perform to the best of their capabilities. Intrinsic motivation comes from within an athlete such as the athlete's desire to set a personal record. Michael Phelps's tenacity and desire to continue engaging in swimming competition despite his record-breaking success and Olympic medals is the epitome of intrinsic motivation. Extrinsic motivation comes from an outside source such as a multimillion-dollar contract or the obtainment of a new championship ring. Research on motivation suggests that the nature of the motivation is far less important that the level. Thus, even though we often hear of the beauty of playing a sport for the pure love of the game, performance excellence is not consistently tied to intrinsically motivated behavior.

There is also evidence to suggest that the relationship between personality and athletic performance is interactional in nature and represents a two-way street. That is, sport participation may change an athlete's personality (Wann, 1997). Some positive changes seen in response to athletic success are increases in self-esteem and self-confidence. There are also potential negative consequences to playing sports, such as an increase in aggression and risk taking behaviors (e.g., binge drinking) that are commonly seen in male team sports or depression or esteem issues that can arise in response to athletic failures.

MEASURING PERSONALITY

Within the sport context, professionals employ sport-specific tests of personality as well as those developed for general populations. Importantly, since individuals who participate in sport are normally healthy, pathology-based tests such as the Minnesota Multiphasic Personality Inventory, Second Edition (MMPI-2) usually are avoided in favor of tests that were developed and standardized for healthy individuals. General tests of personality and mood can provide insight into habits and dispositions that characterize the person in and out of sport. As described earlier, the Profile of Mood States is used very commonly as is the State-Trait Anxiety Inventory (STAI) and the NEO Five Factor Inventory (NEO-FFI) personality test. Sport-specific tests such as the Sport Orientation Questionnaire (SOQ) tend to focus narrowly on characteristics that apply to a sport context, such as competitiveness, motivation, toughness, and aggression. Although testing plays an important role in assessing an individual's characteristics and propensities, most professionals caution about using only one or two tests for assessment. Commonly, multiple tests, as well as behavioral observations, and interviews of the individual and significant others (teammates and coaches) combine to make up the complete assessments.

INJURY RISK AND ASSOCIATED PSYCHOLOGICAL TRAITS

Participation in athletics, particularly at a competitive level, is occasionally accompanied by physical injury. These injuries can range from a mild muscle strain to broken bones and worse. In observations among varying levels of sports, some athletes seem to be afflicted by injuries quite regularly, while others manage to avoid the training room altogether. Many physical and environmental factors play a role in the risk of injury, but psychological factors can also play a role in injury incidence and severity. This has led many researchers to investigate which characteristics differentiate these athletes from one another, including factors such as personality, stress reactions, and coping resources.

Personality and Vulnerability to Injury

One's personality is made up of many individual factors, several of which have been examined to determine their role in the incidence of injury in athletes. One prominent construct has been the "Type A" personality pattern, which is characterized by impatience, time-consciousness, hostility, aggressiveness, a high drive for achievement, and competitiveness. The sports injury literature has shown that athletes who express a higher level of these characteristics report more injuries than those who do not. This is particularly true in those sports that require a great deal of running, as these athletes are likely to practice to the point of an overuse injury and continue competing even when they experience considerable pain. Since aggression and anger are a part of the Type A personality mix, these factors have been investigated on their own as well. Although the feelings of anger may be present in varying levels, it is those who direct high levels of anger outward, but not inward, who have an increased injury risk.

One phrase often used in athletics refers to being "tough-minded." Tough-minded characteristics include being strong-willed, self-assured, assertive, and independent. Athletes are often encouraged by coaches, teammates, and others to possess these traits as they believe that doing so will boost their athletic skill and enhance positive results. While this may hold true, it has been found that being tough-minded actually predicts more severe injuries, though it does not affect the frequency. Athletes with this type of attitude probably take greater risks in the playing field, and therefore are in more situations that could result in severe injury. In addition, they are more likely to continue participating even when they feel physical discomfort.

Further, one's locus of control (i.e., one's belief about personal versus external control over the good and bad results in life) contributes to injury risk. In general, athletes who possess a high external locus of control are at higher risk for incurring more frequent and more severe injuries than those who express an internal locus.

Trait anxiety, or an individual's dispositional level of worry and fear, can manifest in mental, emotional, and physical components. High levels of trait anxiety, especially when the athlete believes it can have a detrimental effect on their performance, places the individual at a greater risk of experiencing an injury. Indeed, it appears that one's injury potential can be the outcome of a self-fulfilling prophecy. Overall, high trait anxiety is significantly related to injury occurrence, while anger, tension, and negative overall mood contribute to the severity of the injury. A negative overall mood state, including depression, general negativity, and hostility, likely contribute to increased muscle tension and fatigue—characteristics that promote the relationship between stress and injury. In contrast, positive mind states such as staying focused, keeping relaxed, and sharing experiences with others have been associated with fewer injuries.

Stress and Injury Risk

In addition to these more stable personality factors, stress has been shown to play a significant role in injury incidence. Most of the research has focused on the occurrence of stressful life events, such as the loss of a loved one, the breakup of a relationship, or moving from one place to another. High levels of life stress over the course of a year have been shown to be associated with a higher incidence of athletic injury, while lower levels were associated with less frequent injury. In essence, the level of life stress seems to be proportional to the occurrence of injury. As Williams and Anderson (1998) have summarized, the majority of studies have indicated that the association is most distinct when the reported life stressors were considered to have a negative influence, but some evidence suggests that previously positive events can also have a negative effect on later injury. Examples of this would be the change of playing status or receipt of awards that later put more pressure on the athlete.

Beyond these larger events, daily hassles are also influential. Though they may not seem as significant initially, consistent daily problems can impact injury vulnerability just as much as major life stress. Specifically, some athletes have been found to experience an increase in daily stressors a week before and the week of incurring an injury. While this association is not as strongly supported as the role of life stress, evidence does indicate an association between these factors.

So why does stress play a role? It has been hypothesized that the physiological response to stress, or the physical changes that result from enduring stress, actually increase the risk of injury. Some of these factors have been shown to occur in times of high stress, such as elevating the athlete's level of anxiety, narrowing of the peripheral visual field, greater distractibility, and slowed reaction time. Studies have shown that performing in stressful situations causes these symptoms to become more prevalent, but these effects are even more pronounced when an individual has experienced high levels of life stress in the last year.

Coping Skills and Injury Potential

Coping resources such as social support, stress management, and general coping behaviors also have a role in injury occurrence. Coping is closely tied with the role of stress, and there is increasing evidence to show that groups of athletes who experience injuries have significantly fewer coping resources as compared to those without injury. Those with a higher level of coping resources are better able to manage stress in adaptive ways, and have greater social support. Social support, or knowing that people love, care, and value us, appears to have a protective role, while a lack of this support can exacerbate the negative effects contributed by stress and therefore lead to higher injury occurrence.

Cognitive skills and behavioral patterns, which are important to coping or effectively managing stress, may also be associated with a greater injury risk. In particular, attentional style has been a good predictor of athletes who get injured. There are sparse data linking other cognitive skills with athletic injury. For example, it may be intuitive to think that athletes' ability to think rationally during stress may influence their potential to become injured; however, the verdict is still out. One thing is certain: the study of coping and injury, although gaining momentum, has many open questions.

INFLUENCE OF PERSONALITY ON RECOVERY AND REHABILITATION

Although the physical consequences of an athletic injury may be obvious, the impact on one's psychological functioning may be subtle and readily missed by coaches, athletes, and even certified athletic trainers (ATCs). However, it is essential to understand both the personal attributes and qualities that athletes espouse before and after an injury as this may influence their physical recovery. Although models of sports rehabilitation have been well established, there is less scientific knowledge regarding the association between personality and lingering symptoms. One such example is the notion of the "*miserable minority*," a small cluster of people who complain of persisting concussive symptoms much longer than others who sustain the same injury. This group has captured the attention of many researchers as they exemplify that for some, a mild traumatic brain injury may not be so mild at all. In other instances, certain athletes return to athletic play much later than expected or even have difficulties adhering to rehabilitation programs. The underlying mechanisms for these phenomena are not yet clearly understood. Could it be that personality features and negative psychological reactions in response to injury are the culprit in some cases? This section focuses on how personality may either positively or negatively influence recovery from athletic injuries and adherence to sports rehabilitation.

An athlete's recovery is both physical and psychological in nature. However, the concept that recovery involves psychological processes is relatively newer and may take secondary priority during initial diagnosis and goal implementation of rehabilitation. The previous section highlighted the large body of scientific literature dedicated to personality and injury potential in recent decades. Can these same traits also predict physical or cognitive recovery from athletic injuries? This is a question that remains largely unanswered. Within the athletic training literature, there has been increasing emphasis on evaluation of the unique psychological perspective that an athlete brings into the injury dynamic and how stress, coping behaviors, and return-to-play issues influence recovery and compliance. It is also widely accepted that psychological factors such as stress, depression, and anxiety can lead to nervous system dysregulation (e.g., increased heart rate); chronic stress responses in the body (e.g., elevation of cortisol and other stress hormones); and reduced immune system functions, which are vital to the physical recovery process. Generally speaking, anxiety, coping resources, and other specific traits in athletes associated with greater injury risk probably factor into length of recovery as well. For example, as mentioned previously, athletes with a "Type A" personality may continue playing despite experiencing an injury, thereby taking longer to heal. Moreover, athletes who engage in more risky behaviors, such as drinking alcohol excessively, "partying," and getting little sleep, may experience slower physical recoveries. More specifically, within the context of concussions, recent evidence suggests that a history of learning and attentional difficulties, as well as behavioral problems (mostly in children and adolescents) may lead to more persisting symptoms. Thus, identifying athletes who have reduced psychological adjustment in the early phases of recovery and implementing appropriate rehabilitation interventions to combat the persisting symptoms is paramount.

Just as personality may influence injury potential and recovery, the physical injury can also negatively impact an athlete's psychological functioning. In a comprehensive literature review, Roh and Perna (2000) found that 90 percent of studies showed that both male and female athletes at varying competitive levels across both contact and noncontact sports exhibit significant psychological distress (e.g., depression, anxiety, anger) in response to athletic injury. This is reasonable to expect as sports injuries can dramatically interfere with an individual's lifestyle, particularly if he or she is a highly competitive collegiate or professional athlete. For example, an injury can shift and change one's social interactions with coaches and teammates, activities (e.g., attending practices and games), ability to exercise, and even earning potential. For these reasons, we propose that more severe injuries have a greater potential to negatively impact one's emotional status due to the consequences associated with them. For example, an anterior cruciate ligament (ACL) tear or rotator cuff injury will require longer time away from a sport in comparison to a minor ankle sprain that takes weeks to heal. More severe injuries may also involve more medical management (e.g., surgery, medication, longer rehabilitation program), which may lead to psychological maladjustment.

Even with seemingly minor injuries, the significance of an injury to an athlete should be understood within a developmental context. That is, the athlete's perspective on an injury will differ in terms of their age, talent, and need for athletic prowess as part of their identity and sense of self-worth. For example, a competitive high school athlete may depend on sports participation for validation by their peers or may easily lose confidence in his or her athletic abilities, while a professional athlete may minimize symptoms in order to continue playing and may misinterpret that their talent will overcome their pain. They may also want to be viewed as "tough" by coaches, teammates, and sports fans. For example, Eric Lindros continued to play professional hockey through multiple concussions, pain, and a great deal of emotional turmoil. Quite likely, the desire to be seen as "tough" played a major role in his behavior. Thus, it is pertinent that ATCs and other professionals make referrals for psychotherapy, when deemed appropriate. Psychological interventions aimed at improving adjustment to athletic injury (discussed shortly) may be essential to the overall recovery process.

Indeed, an athlete's beliefs about injuries and personal characteristics may also play a role in their initial reporting of injuries (i.e., the first step toward rehabilitation adherence) as well as compliance with the various phases of sports rehabilitation. This is an often-neglected area in scientific investigations, particularly in respect to personality, which may be due to the misconception that athletes, unlike other rehabilitation patients, may be more compliant with trainers due to their inherent "personality" of being tough-minded, competitive, and highly motivated. To the contrary, problems do frequently arise such as athletes being overzealous to return to play too soon or being under-motivated to participate in rehabilitation or go back on the field. It is reasonable to expect that asking athletes to put themselves through "blood, sweat, and tears" for a substantial amount of time would lead to issues with complying with medical professionals' requests. Additionally, athletes with depression may pose a greater risk for poor adherence as data from the general medical literature demonstrate that depressed patients are three times more likely to be noncompliant with medical advice.

Unique factors and personality traits may aid in sports rehabilitation compliance. Some examples are greater social support; higher pain tolerance; higher self-motivation; and greater goal-directed behavior. A history of being previously injured is also associated with better compliance with rehabilitation exercises, which may be explained by learned coping behaviors. Wiese, Weiss, and Yukelson (1991) also discovered that athletic trainers perceived better coping and adherence by athletes when they exhibited greater listening skills, positive attitude, intrinsic motivation, and willingness to learn about the rehabilitation techniques. In general, it is a reasonable assumption that athletes will adhere to training and medical staff requests when the desire to return to play outweighs any reinforcers to stay away from the game (e.g., the highly competitive player who does not want to lose his or her starting position).

Personality factors may also lead to noncompliance with sports rehabilitation. For example, those who experience physical complaints associated with anxiety (e.g., headaches, stomachaches) may experience greater sensitivity to physical changes associated with their injury and may be less inclined to fight through these symptoms in rehabilitation sessions. Additionally, it is well known that those who internalize anxiety may be more easily distracted than their peers and may miss important cues in their environment. This may result in athletes being less focused during sessions or missing important information that leads to suboptimal rehabilitation. In a broad sense, anxiety may impede rehabilitation as these athletes may not trust their trainer or believe the "evidence" that they are fully recovered when they are cleared to play. Instead, they may have excessive fear of returning to play or may fear getting reinjured, which can act as a strong motivator in not complying with rehabilitation. Similarly, athletes who are depressed, exhibit low self-esteem, or who lack coping skills may not respond well to obstacles such as a physical injury, which could impede their motivation to persist through their pain. In general, athletes who find reinforcers for continuing in rehabilitation rather than returning to athletic play (e.g., a bench player who gains sympathy from a coach and/or teammates) may experience less motivation and be less compliant with rehabilitation.

Although an athlete who is determined to return to play in a short time period may be viewed positively by spectators (and coaches), there are some potential negatives in the sports rehabilitation environment. Tough-minded athletes may not tell ATCs when they experience pain during rehabilitation. In general, athletes whose identities are strongly intertwined with sports may exhibit an "I have nothing left to lose" or "no pain, no gain" mentality. As a result, these athletes may push themselves to their physical limits, experience increased pain, and may have a slowed rather than quick recovery with a greater potential to do more harm than good.

PSYCHOLOGICAL ADJUSTMENT TO ATHLETIC INJURY AND INTERVENTIONS

The way in which an athlete responds to injury and the way in which they will adjust to any new complications within their team and the sports rehabilitation environment can be unpredictable. As described throughout this chapter, consideration of what the athlete was like before the injury (personality, coping ability) as well as external stressors (stressful live events and situational stressors outside of the injury) is paramount as they can influence an athlete's response to an injury. In addition to evaluating prior psychological traits, there are numerous psychological effects of an injury itself, including anxiety, fear, stress, identity loss, depression, anger, and loss of confidence, which may require psychological interventions. An athlete who more strongly identifies with their athletic role may experience more emotional distress in response to an injury than an athlete who does not strongly identify with their athletic role. Due to the relationship that coaches, trainers, and physicians have with injured players, they represent the first line of defense against poor adjustment. Their identification of changes to athletes' mood states and seeking appropriate referrals to a psychologist is essential. In this upcoming portion of the chapter, we will demonstrate the way in which a psychologist can act as a liaison between athletes, coaches, and ATCs and implement effective therapeutic interventions with athletes.

Family, Team, and Coaching Dynamics

Level of perceived social support plays an important role in an athlete's psychological adjustment to an injury. Psychologists may need to actively advocate on behalf of the athlete, and they can consult with relatives, teammates, and coaches to ensure that their psychological needs are a top priority. For example, it may be appropriate to provide family members with knowledge of the physical injury and potentially negative psychological reactions to injury early on in a general way so that their fears or frustrations do not exacerbate the athlete's stress level or anxiety. Relatives can improve an athlete's self-esteem by clarifying strengths that he or she exhibits outside of sports. They can propose alternative activities so that the athlete can continue to enjoy themselves and not just focus on returning to play.

Teammates and coaches also provide a vital supportive role in the rehabilitation process as they enable the athlete to stay connected to their athletic identity. When an athlete is sidelined due to an injury, he or she is not able to fully interact with teammates, which may lead to feelings of social isolation. Thus, athletes should be encouraged to continue to attend practice and travel to games so that they can continue to feel as if they are part of the "team." Athletes will also take cues from their coaches regarding how to interpret their injury and how to appropriately cope with the situation. A coach's response to an athlete's injury can also impact adherence to rehabilitation. It needs to be communicated to coaches that pressuring their player to return back to play too soon may negatively impact their recovery. On the other hand, coaches who only pay attention to bench players when they are hurt may in fact increase the athlete's desire to stay in rehabilitation. Moreover, coaches who ignore injured players may lead them to feel less motivated to return to play.

Psychology in the Athletic Training Environment

How the athlete's athletic trainer reacts to his or her injury and their approach to sports rehabilitation will impact their coping. Athletes who are goal-directed may do well when rehabilitation is conducted within a sports context so that they can imagine themselves better developing as an athlete. Areas of athletic weakness in their sport prior to the injury can also be targeted. For example, a basketball player who tears her anterior cruciate ligament (ACL) may focus on dribbling drills to improve her potential to play a guard position upon returning to play. A football player can work on upper body strength when experiencing an ankle injury. This helps the athlete maintain a mentality they had while playing their respective sport, where they can find ways to improve themselves in the sports arena, not only in terms of their physical recovery. Athletes who are highly motivated and competitive may also respond to athletic trainers who focus on the mental intensity of the sport while in a rehabilitation session. This may involve strategies such as "Yesterday I saw you complete two sets; I bet you can do three sets today." Obviously, these strategies need to be applied in a reasonable manner. Athletic trainers can also conduct rehabilitation exercises within the context of their practices. For example, the athlete can participate in bicycle exercises while watching practice or may even engage in a walk-through of game plays in a less rigorous fashion.

Psychological Interventions with Athletes

Sports psychologists employ a variety of counseling techniques with athletes such as relaxation, imagery, cognitive restructuring, goal setting, and modeling. There are multiple forms of relaxation, such as yoga, breathing techniques, and meditation. Relaxation allows the athlete to become aware of his or her body in order to reduce stress. It is common for relaxation techniques to be combined with visual imagery. Visual imagery requires athletes to (a) imagine that they can both see and feel the injury healing; (b) engage in thinking about being recovered and injury free; and (c) imagine performing at their best. Cognitive restructuring aims at teaching athletes to replace their negative self-talk, (e.g., "I am never going to heal") with positive self-talk (e.g., "I am going to be healed and back on the court before I know it!"). Positive self-talk allows the athlete to focus on improving rather than on engaging in a defeatist's attitude. Goal setting is also important as evidence suggests that those who set goals heal faster than those who did not set goals. This requires athletes to think of goals; imagine meeting those goals; and imagine feelings associated with these accomplishments. Finally, modeling is another useful technique as it allows athletes to realize that other people who were in a similar situation as them were able to recover or make progress, and that they, too, will be able to recover.

CONCLUSIONS AND TAKE-HOME MESSAGES

The study of personality factors in sports psychology has focused historically on the many potential relationships between personality and ability, sport performance, sport suitability, injury risk, and rehabilitation potential. Although many plausible theories have been proposed to relate these factors, the best-researched and empirically validated relationships have been found to relate injury and injury-recovery risk to a few psychological and personality variables. Specifically, level of life stress and type and extent of coping skills are key factors in predicting injury and recovery in athletes. Future efforts are likely to focus on more traditional personality factors such as extraversion, neuroticism, and the like. There also is a developing theme of using personality tests to select individuals for specific sports and teams. No body of research has validated such efforts to date. In summary, although personality approaches are attractive and intuitive ways to understand an athlete in a competitive setting, underlying traits are seen at best as only partially contributing to the variability in performance. The social setting, the reinforcing community, and the athlete's phenomenological appreciation of the situation contribute at least as much to predictions of performance and self-satisfaction.

RECOMMENDED READING

DiMatteo, M. R., Lepper, H. S., & Croghan, T. W. (2000). Depression is a risk factor for noncompliance with medical treatment. *Archives of Internal Medicine*, 160, 2101–2107.

Ekenman, I., Hassmen, P., Koivula, N., Rolf, C., & Fellander-Tsai, L. (2001). Stress fractures of the tibia: Can personality traits help us detect the injury-prone athlete? *Scandinavian Journal of Medicine and Science in Sports*, 11, 87–95.

Lavallee, L., & Flint, F. (1996). The relationship of stress, competitive anxiety, mood state, and social support to athletic injury. *Journal of Athletic Training*, 31, 296–299.

Pargman, D. (1993). *Psychological Bases of Sport Injuries*. Morgantown, WV: Fitness Information Technology, Inc.

Wann, D. L. (1997). *Sport Psychology*. Upper Saddle River, New Jersey: Prentice Hall.

REFERENCES

Andersen, M. B., & Williams, J. M. (1993). Psychological risk factors and injury prevention. In J. Heil (Ed.), *Psychology of sport injury* (pp. 49–55). Champaign, IL: Human Kinetics.

Ben-Ari, R., Tsur, Y., & Har-Even, D. (2006). Procedural justice, stress appraisal, and athletes' attitudes. *International Journal of Stress Management*, 13, 23–44.

Carney, R. M., Freedland, K. E., & Veith, R. C. (2005). *Psychosomatic Medicine*, 67, 29–33.

Collins, M. W., Grindel, S. H., Lovell, M. R., Dede, D. E., Moser, D. J., Phalin, B. R., et al. (1999). Relationship between concussion and neuropsychological performance in college football players. *JAMA*, 282, 964–970.

Cooper, L. (1969) Athletics, activity and personality: A review of the literature. *Research Quarterly*, 40, 17–22.

Johnson, R. C., & Rosen, L. A. (2000). Sports behavior of ADHD children. *Journal of Attention Disorders*, 4, 150–160.

Levin, H. S., Hanten, G., Max, J., Xiaoqi, L., Swank, P., Ewing-Cobbs, L., et al. (2007). Symptoms of attention-deficit/hyperactivity disorder following traumatic brain injury in children. *Journal of Developmental and Behavioral Pediatrics*, 28, 108–118.

Martens, R. (1975). *Social psychology and physical activity*. New York: Harper & Row.

Milne, M., Hall, C., Forwell, L. (2005). Self-efficacy, imagery use, and adherence to rehabilitation by injured athletes.*Journal of Sports Rehabilitation*, 14, 150.

Morgan, W. (1979). Prediction of performance in athletics. In P. Klavora and J. W. Daniel, Eds., *Coach, athlete and the sport psychologist*. Champaign, IL: Human Kinetics.

Ray, R., & Wiese-Bjornstal, D. M. (1999). *Counseling in sports medicine*. Champaign, IL: Human Kinetics Publishers.

Reiche, E. M., Nunes, S. O., & Morimoto, H. K. (2004). Stress, depression, the immune system, and cancer. *Lancet Oncology*, 5, 617–625.

Roh, J. L., & Perna, F. M. (2000). Psychology/counseling: A universal competency in athletic training. *Journal of Athletic Training*, 35, 458–465.

Rowley, A. J., Landers, D. M., Kyllo, L. B., & Etnier, J. L. (1995). Does the iceberg profile discriminate between successful and less successful athletes? A meta-analysis. *Journal of Sport & Exercise Psychology*, 17, 185–199.

Sport Psychologist, 5, 25–40.

Thompson, N. J., & Morris, R. D. (1994). Predicting injury risk in adolescent football players: The importance of psychological variables. *Journal of Pediatric Psychology*, 19, 415–429.

Wiese, D. M., Weiss, M. R., & Yukelson, D. P. (1991). Sport psychology in the training room: A survey of athletic trainers.*The Sport Psychologist*, 5, 15–25.

Williams, J. M., & Andersen, M. B. (1998). Psychosocial antecedents of sport injury: Review and critique of the stress and injury model. *Journal of Applied Sport Psychology*, 10, 5–25.

Williams, J. M., Hogan, T. D., & Andersen, M. B. (1993). Positive states of mind and athletic injury risk. *Psychosomatic Medicine*, 55, 468–472.

Wittig, A. F., & Schurr, K. T. (1994). Psychological characteristics of woman volleyball players: Relationships with injuries, rehabilitation, and team success. *Personality and Social Psychology Bulletin*, 20, 322–330.

Chapter 6

The Psychological Aspects of Sports-related Injuries

Stephen A. Russo and Susana Quintana Marikle

Given the number of injuries people sustain while participating in sport and exercise, it is little wonder that a significant amount of psychological research has been devoted to understanding the ramifications of these injuries. It is estimated that as many as 17 million people are injured each year in sport and exercise-related activities, which provides more-than-sufficient justification for the need for continued exploration into this area. This chapter focuses on the psychological aspects of injuries sustained during sport and athletic activities. For both the athletes that sustain sports-related injuries as well as the sports medicine professionals that treat these individuals, having an understanding of the current knowledge base in this area is paramount. Not only does this information help us understand the typical athlete's response to injury, but possessing this information can also have a tremendous impact on the course, progression, and ultimate outcome of the physical injuries that are sustained in sports.

FREQUENCY AND TIMING OF ATHLETIC INJURIES

Athletes of all ages run some risk of sustaining injuries, from minor to severe. In most cases, several factors are involved when determining both the risk of an injury as well as what elements are relevant to the athlete's eventual recovery. According to the Centers for Disease

Control, sport- and recreation-related injuries comprise close to 50 percent of emergency room visits among individuals 15 to 19 years of age and, as staggering as this number already is, it does not account for the injuries that do not lead to an emergency room visit. Given that many injuries go unreported, it is extremely difficult to estimate the true number of injuries that occur while people are engaging in athletic activities. To compound matters further, the psychological concepts of "walking it off" or "playing through" an injury are among the most often-cited sport clichés, making individuals even more reluctant to seek medical treatment when injury occurs on the field of play. This mentality, though pervasive in sports, is not conducive to seeking appropriate medical assistance and often contributes to an individual's reluctance to seek help, particularly when the precipitating event is perceived by the individual to be a "minor" injury.

When studying U.S. high school student-athletes participating in practice or competition across nine sports, the CDC estimated that 1,442,533 injuries occur at a rate of 2.4 injuries per 1,000 "athletic exposures," where "athletic exposures" refers to every time an athlete practices, competes, or engages in some form of organized athletic training routine. The CDC noted that the highest injury rate occurred in football, which had 4.36 injuries per 1,000 athlete exposures, and was followed by wrestling (2.50), boys' and girls' soccer (2.43 and 2.36, respectively), and girls' basketball (2.01). At the other end of the spectrum, boys' basketball, volleyball, baseball, and softball all had injury rates of fewer than 2.0 injuries per 1,000 athlete exposures. Overall, sprains, strains, and other impairments to the lower extremities account for the majority of sport-related injuries, regardless of the sport being played and whether the injury was sustained during competition or practice. Thus, it appears that all sport participants incur some risk of injury due to the similar movements associated with their practice activities and training regimens. In a study of high school athletes across a variety of sports, the sport in question, the gender of the participant, as well as whether the individual had suffered a previous injury were also related to the incidence of injury (Rechel, Yard, & Comstock, 2008). Other factors such as grade level, participation in multiple sports, years of playing experience, and body mass index (BMI, often used as an estimate of fitness) were also found to play a role in varsity sport injuries (Knowles, Marshall, Bowling, Loomis, Millikan, Yang, et al, 2006).

While all athletes expose themselves to risk of injury through their practice and training regimens, it seems that the timing of the season and the intensity of the activity may be related to the occurrence of injury. For example, some researchers have found that preseason injuries are significantly more common than those sustained in-season, postseason, or during practice, suggesting that perhaps a lack of conditioning or a sudden change in the intensity and/or quality of training is associated with injury. Conversely, some authors have found that competition, not practice, results in higher rates of injury and greater ratios of head, face, and neck injuries as well as more concussions and other more severe types of problems. The increase in injury rates during competition is supported by a CDC study in which injury rates were found to be higher in competition than they were during practice across nine sports. Finally, in a 16-year study of collegiate injuries across 15 sports, it was found that athletes were significantly more likely to sustain an injury during competition than during practice. Thus, it appears that intensity of activity may be associated with injury, as the increased incidence of injury during competition could be attributable to the increased effort, increased contact (legal and illegal), and increased exposure to risky behaviors that typically occur under most game conditions.

UNDERSTANDING COMMON REACTIONS TO ATHLETIC INJURY

For individuals who participate in athletics and sport-related activities on a regular basis, injury can be a stressful and life-altering experience. While the physical ramifications and ultimate prognoses vary according to the severity, type, and location of the injury, many athletes experience emotional upheaval both immediately following an injury as well as during the rehabilitation process. For example, a study by Brewer and Petrie (2002) reported that as many as 24 percent of athletes report significant emotional difficulties such as depression or anxiety following injury, particularly in the first 4 to 8 weeks after the injury occurs. Thus, injury can influence the emotional state of an athlete and can challenge athletes at all levels to cope with an unforeseen stressor. Concerns about the severity of the injury and the length of the rehabilitation process frequently occur, and athletes may also become frustrated with inactivity or overly focused on the pain sensations they experience throughout treatment. In addition to injury-specific worries, athletes may also doubt whether they will ever fully recover or may become concerned about whether they will return to their pre-injury level of play. Fears of being reinjured upon returning to practice or being permanently replaced by a teammate are other common concerns following injury. In a study of adolescent athletes, it was found that this kind of distress persisted even after athletes had physically recuperated from their injuries (Newcomer & Perna, 2003), suggesting that younger athletes may be especially sensitive to injury-related trauma and may also be at increased risk for developing long-term problems following their sports-related injuries.

Stage Models

Recognizing the psychological or emotional impact of injury is important because an athlete's ability to cope with injury-related stress can influence their adherence to the rehabilitation process and might be the difference between their successful or unsuccessful completion of treatment. Given that rehabilitation outcomes have a direct impact on athletic performance, return-to-play issues, and various aspects of an athlete's life outside of sports, it's important for both athletes and the health care providers that treat them to be aware of their emotional state. To understand what an athlete encounters psychologically once they become injured, some clinicians have used "stage" models of bereavement as a conceptual foundation for research, intervention, and clinical management purposes. A number of stage theories are in existence, primarily because an injury can represent a great "loss" in an athlete's life, but the model that has received the most significant attention was the one proposed by Kubler-Ross (1969) in her seminal book, *On death and dying*. Essentially, the Kubler-Ross model focuses on the psychological response of losing a loved one; but when adapted, it suggests that athletes respond to the "loss" of their athletic status similarly to the way a person responds to the death of a loved individual. The model consists of five basic stages (denial, anger, bargaining, depression, and acceptance) and has, historically, been one of the more commonly reported psychological theories regarding athletic injury. According to this and other stage theories, injured athletes are thought to pass through a preordained and systematic progression of psychological reactions as they face the emotional aspects of their injury and their recovery.

Although stage theories are functional models that make intuitive sense, they often fail to address personal or contextual factors that are unique to individual athletes, such as social support systems, personality factors, or life experiences. Moreover, they have not been consistently supported in research on athletic injuries because athletes' reactions are inherently varied and their responses generally do not follow a set pattern. For example, whereas one athlete may deny the severity of a knee injury and cycle between anger and depression before fully committing to the rehabilitation process, an athlete with a similar injury may completely circumvent any form of emotional distress and readily accept the information provided by the treatment team, thus beginning the rehabilitation process with less hesitation and uncertainty.

Cognitive Models

Other psychological injury models have focused on cognitions and the impact that an athlete's thoughts and perceptions can have on their emotional response to injury. In particular, cognitive appraisals, or the instinctive process where people critically evaluate their capacity to meet the demands of a given situation, have garnered a considerable amount of attention. The most renowned cognitive model is an "integrative model" promoted by Wiese-Bjornstal, Smith, Shaffer, and Morrey (1998) that also incorporates personal and situational factors into an understanding of injured athletes' psychological reactions. At the center of this (and other) cognitive models is the notion that what an athlete thinks about his or her injury as well as how they interpret their injury, their goals, and their rehabilitation program can have a significant impact on their long-term outcomes. Personal factors such as one's tendency to appraise an event as either positive or negative, the perceived intensity of the stressor, and the individual's instinctive coping style are crucially important when evaluating an athlete's coping process. Also related is the source of the individual's stress as well as the characteristics of the sporting event. Thus, thought patterns appear to have an important impact on an athlete's psychological reaction to injury because they influence the athlete's emotional state as well as their commitment to a prescribed rehabilitation program.

The pervasive influence of cognitions and cognitive appraisals has been documented in both an athlete's emotional reaction to injury as well as their eventual compliance with the rehabilitation process. The appraisal process appears to be so meaningful because, at its basic level, cognitive appraisals represent how an athlete evaluates his or her current situation and interprets the meaning of a multitude of variables and characteristics associated with their injury. While an individual's background, personality, and preexisting level of functioning may influence their general cognitive style, attributions following injury appear to take on greater power and influence due to the heightened levels of stress and uncertainty that invariably follow athletic injury. In essence, athletes make evaluations and interpretations about factors such as the reason they were injured, the severity of their injury, and the level of performance they eventually hope to obtain. More importantly, athletes make internal cognitive assessments about whether they are capable of overcoming the obstacles they now face or accomplishing the athletic goals they have set for themselves. This process has both direct and indirect influence on their treatment compliance and their emotional response. Professionals who care for athletes following injury must recognize the influence of these cognitive processes, as cognitions and cognitive appraisals can foster either effective or ineffective coping strategies on the part of injured athletes. For example, if an athlete doubts that they are capable of returning to play quickly, they may be less likely to complete a daily stretching program that is outlined by the medical team. Conversely, if an athlete believes they are a "fast healer," they may be more inclined to complete their prescribed daily exercise regimen or comply with the athletic limitations imposed by their medical professionals.

Personal and Situational Characteristics

Injuries do not happen in a vacuum, and an athlete's strengths and coping style are particularly relevant to his or her individual response to injury. For example, it has been found that ineffective coping to a given stressor can lead to negative outcomes, such as when increased muscle tension or muscular "bracing" of an injured area is persistently used to reduce pain sensations but ultimately leads to a reduced range of motion in the affected joint. The effectiveness of an athlete's coping response to a serious injury is often influenced by their perceptions of the injury, how much they identify with the role of being an athlete, and their perceived progress in rehabilitation. From a psychological perspective, anxiety and depression are common reactions to stressful events such as injury, with some people describing these temporary emotional states in athletes as "adjustment reactions." Emotional disturbances of this form are frequently reported in the early phases of the rehabilitation process and do not constitute "abnormal" emotional functioning unless the emotional reaction persists beyond the initial adjustment period or begins to interfere with the rehabilitation process.

The anxiety associated with injury for athletes encompasses worry about playing status, fear of the possibility of reinjury, and concerns regarding whether they will make a full recovery. Depressive symptoms are common as well, as injured athletes have been found to have a greater proportion of negative emotions when compared to their noninjured peers and a significant proportion of athletes feel a perceived pressure to ignore physical problems. Less common are the more severe emotional reactions that can follow gruesome or extreme injuries. Athletes who experience particularly gruesome injuries (such as a compound fracture where the broken bone can protrude from the skin) can experience the proceedings as traumatic events, with the injury potentially leading to the development of Posttraumatic Stress Disorder (PTSD). However, in order for this diagnosis to be given, individuals must encounter a particularly harrowing event, in which they fear that they or another individual is going to die, and experience significant interference in their social or occupational lives for well over a month after the injury occurs. Indeed, this kind of response to an athletic injury is rare, but readers should recognize that many athletic injuries could qualify as a "traumatic" experience.

Often times, the athlete's personal characteristics and the circumstances that surround the injury have a direct and indirect impact on their emotional reaction. In his review of the literature, Brewer (2001) noted that older athletes, those with greater psychological investment in playing professional sports, and those with a more pessimistic attitude experienced greater emotional disturbance following significant injury. When studying the role of gender in the experiences of injured collegiate athletes, Granito (2002) found that female athletes were more likely to report greater negative experiences with their coaches than male athletes (94% compared to 20%, respectively), and female athletes were also more likely to express concern over how the injury would affect their future physical health. Conversely, male athletes were more likely than female athletes to mention the support of a significant other during the rehabilitation process. Situational characteristics such as injury severity (i.e., the amount of impairment that an injury causes on daily activities as well as sport performance), and the prognosis and complexity of the entire recovery process have also been associated with greater emotional disturbance in athletes following injury.

REHABILITATION ISSUES FOLLOWING ATHLETIC INJURIES

Once injured, athletes typically engage in a number of musculoskeletal interventions in order to promote a successful return to regular training and competitive play. As noted in Brewer's (2001) review, it is not uncommon for athletes to engage in a variety of activities during their physical rehabilitation. As this is a psychological review, the following list is not meant to be an exhaustive review of physical therapy intervention strategies. If readers are interested in reading a more comprehensive review of rehabilitation interventions, they are encouraged to review any number of readings on the subject and may find it beneficial to begin with Brewer's (2001) review.

Typically, activity levels are modified and/or significantly reduced during the initial recovery period, as rest is often used as a way to promote physical healing. This is particularly true if a surgical intervention is required to correct an injury. Although the specific rehabilitation regimen varies greatly, depending on the type, form, severity, and location of the injury, physical rehabilitation can include some form of musculoskeletal bracing or taping procedures as well as any number of therapeutic modalities. Stretching and strengthening exercises, which can consist of passive stretching, manual resistance, or mechanical resistance exercises, can be coordinated through either an athletic trainer or physical therapy professional under the direction of a primary care physician or team doctor. Moreover, it is not uncommon for athletes to take medications to reduce pain and swelling. Functional activities, which include both activities of daily living as well as sport-specific movements, are often targeted during the rehabilitation process, and modalities such as hot/cold packs, ultrasound, electrical stimulation, whirlpools, massage, iontophoresis, and other techniques are used in conjunction with any or all of the aforementioned interventions.

Although physical rehabilitation is often viewed as a structured and straightforward process, it should be noted that athletes may often encounter a number of physical and psychological challenges during this time period. For example, it is not uncommon for athletes to become discouraged by the physical limitations associated with their injury, particularly if they compare their post-injury functioning to their pre-injury level of ability. Because physical rehabilitation is, essentially, the systematic improvement in one's physical functioning, it frequently requires individuals to endure pain and discomfort while they attempt to improve their body's capabilities. This process takes time, perseverance, and discipline on the part of the individual and, for athletes, frequently involves frustration over the pace and timing of their recovery. When athletes inherently try to "push through" their physical limitations at a pace they are accustomed to, it can result in increased pain, swelling, and discomfort as well as significant setbacks in the recovery process or, at worst, additional injuries. Thus, it is important for athletes to understand their injuries and comply with the treatment plan outlined by their medical providers. Conversely, treatment providers must be on the lookout for the warning signs described earlier that indicate an athlete is not coping with the emotional and psychological aspects of their rehabilitation in an ideal manner. Specifically, an athlete's emotional state and their thought processes should be evaluated regularly to determine if their mental recovery is enhancing their physical rehabilitation or is actually interfering with it.

Personal and Contextual Influences on Rehabilitation

The athlete's level of consistency in engaging in treatment and their ultimate compliance with the prescribed treatment process is perhaps more important than the specific type of rehabilitation performed. Similar to the research on an athlete's psychological reaction to injury, it appears that both personal and situational factors contribute to treatment compliance in an athletic population. As previously mentioned, the level of emotional disturbance associated with an injury's onset is frequently associated with reduced levels of adherence. In addition, frustration, anxiety, and disenchantment with either the care providers or the outlined treatment plan appear to have a negative impact on an athlete's compliance with treatment. Conversely, a high level of pain tolerance, expectations of positive treatment outcome, and an internal locus of control are associated with improved rehabilitation adherence. To that end, psychological resilience has been demonstrated in both physical and psychological contexts, and a number of authors have identified protective psychological traits that allow individuals to overcome difficulties with relatively greater ease. Qualities such as tough-mindedness and the psychological concept of hardiness (which is explained below) have associated with resilience in a variety of settings and appear to be particularly influential in athletic populations where recovery from injury is important.

Associated with self-confidence, hardiness represents a trait that is crucial to a person's resilient response to injury because, at its core, it is the ability to maintain a positive attitude and see difficult situations as more challenging and less threatening. Individuals with high levels of hardiness believe they can have a positive influence on their surroundings and can learn from both the positive as well as the negative events they experience in their lives. As a result, hardy individuals experience less distress and are able to maintain a sense of commitment and purpose in their daily lives, even when circumstances are less than ideal. For example, elite-level athletes appear to have higher levels of overall hardiness when compared to less accomplished athletes as well as the general population. Generally, hardy athletes tend to respond to stressful situations in a more positive, calm, and confident manner than individuals who are less hardy. And since the hardy individual's capacity to absorb extreme levels of stress without suffering debilitating effects is higher than most people's ability, it is expected that these individuals would handle the process of recovering from injury with less difficulty.

The factors listed above help "hardy" individuals adhere to the demands of a difficult physical rehabilitation regimen to a greater degree. Other qualities, such as the presence of positive emotion and positive attributions about the rehabilitation process, have also been associated with greater treatment compliance. In other words, individuals who endure physical and emotional discomfort more effectively and have higher expectations for themselves, including positive expectations of their ability to successfully complete a rehabilitation program, show greater treatment compliance.

From a contextual standpoint, a number of factors are associated with increased levels of rehabilitation adherence. Factors that are likely to improve an athlete's compliance with treatment are the convenience, comfort, and proximity of the rehabilitation facility as well as the perceived amount of time an athlete has to exercise. The relative importance of the treatment process to the athlete, their belief in the efficacy of the treatment plan, and the athlete's perception of the injury severity as well as his or her perceived susceptibility to additional injury or complications without rehabilitation are also influences on an athlete's adherence to rehabilitation.

Social Support

It is important to keep in mind that athletes, typically, are surrounded by people who are invested in their well-being and their overall performance. An injured athlete will often rely on family members, friends, and significant others. When grappling with the emotional aspects of an injury, athletes may also turn to coaches, assistant coaches, athletic trainers, and teammates. Social support from those close to the injured athlete is associated with positive rehabilitation outcomes and serves to help athletes maintain a sense of control over their stressors. However, there must be compatibility between what the injured athlete needs and what the support provider is willing or able to provide. For example, Division I collegiate athletes reported that assistant coaches tend to provide more support pre-injury than during rehabilitation. During rehabilitation, injured athletes were more satisfied with the social support provided by athletic trainers than head or assistant coaches' support, perhaps because these individuals take greater interest in the athlete's actual recovery or are less likely to pressure them to return to the playing field prematurely or view them as being "wimps" because of the pain they report. Also, if an athlete perceived that an individual's support was influential pre-injury, the supportive individual was likely to be perceived as influential to the athlete's well-being during the rehabilitation process. A study of injured high school athletes supports this, noting that athletes who thought their coaches were listening and emotionally supportive during rehabilitation were more influential to their well-being than coaches who only provided support prior to the injury. Thus, listening and emotional support provided during rehabilitation was perceived as more significant than support given before the occurrence of injury. Interestingly, it may not take much to demonstrate such support (e.g., an encouraging phone call or text message, showing genuine interest in the athlete's physical status), but it appears that it is helpful when athletes know their family, friends, coaches, athletic trainers, and teammates are supporting their recovery.

Social support serves to boost the morale, commitment, and attitude of the injured athlete (Brewer, 2001), but it also seems that the importance of social support following injury is partly due to the social nature of athletics. As noted by several authors, the social interactions of injured athletes with coaches, teammates, and other sport personnel change dramatically following their removal from an athletic environment. Social isolation and disconnection from friends, family, and their formerly supportive teammates is not uncommon among athletes following injury, particularly if the athlete ceases to participate in regularly scheduled team activities such as practices or team meetings. In fact, in a study of athletes who sustained season-ending injuries, Gould et al. (1997) noted that using social resources wisely and maintaining a connection to the competitive environment were among the most important suggestions that athletes had for others who were about to endure an extended rehabilitation process.

SUMMARY AND IMPLICATIONS

Unfortunately, injury is an all-too-common experience in athletics. While the true incidence of athletic injury varies according to the sport being played, the situation, and time of athletic season, it can be expected that a significant number athletes will experience some type of injury over the course of their athletic career. Given that the nature and severity of athletic injuries vary greatly, it is difficult to predict how athletes will respond to a sudden change in their athletic status or physical capabilities. However, the notion that all athletes will invariably experience a similar, predetermined emotional progression following athletic injuries has not been supported by the research in this area.

Many factors contribute to an athlete's emotional reaction following injury and their subsequent behavioral response to physical rehabilitation. Since it has been consistently shown that athletes generally experience injury as a stressful event, the post-injury reactions that these individuals demonstrate are often a reflection of their thought processes and coping styles as well as their overall capacity to cope with unpredictable stressors. Thus, an athlete's emotional and psychological functioning prior to injury, their history of injury, and their unique personality will ultimately combine with the characteristics of the injury itself to produce a psychological response. Whereas some athletes will be adequately prepared to cope with the stress associated with injury and physical rehabilitation, it can be anticipated that many athletes will either be overwhelmed by the specifics of the athletic injury or will be woefully unprepared to cope with the psychological ramifications of the event.

Significant emotional reactions immediately following injury appear to be relatively common in athletic populations and, in some situations, these emotional disturbances can persist throughout the recovery process. However, it is generally expected that athletes' emotionality will diminish over the course of their physical recovery and that active coping skills (which is often defined as their compliance with treatment and/or commitment to rehabilitation) will become more prominent over time. In all likelihood, injured athletes will experience varying levels of transient anxiety, depression, or other negative emotions. If the symptoms are prolonged or become worse over time, it is advisable that these athletes seek professional treatment. In addition, based on the information discussed within this chapter, one could anticipate that athletes with certain personality or social characteristics would be at greater risk for developing more significant problems. Examples of these would be injured athletes who are more pessimistic, socially isolated, or less hopeful about themselves, their care providers, or their ability to meet the demands of physical rehabilitation. While these characteristics may not necessarily have a negative impact on an athlete's performance prior to being injured, given the inherent likelihood of injury involved in athletic participation, it may be beneficial for parents, coaches, and medical personnel to recognize and address these characteristics early on in an athlete's playing career so that they are not "at risk" for the development of long-term emotional problems following injury.

An athlete's belief system or, more specifically, their cognitive style appears to have an important influence on both their psychological reactions to injury as well as adherence to a prescribed physical rehabilitation program. It seems that athletes who demonstrate tough-mindedness and positive expectations for recovery are more likely to comply with treatment recommendations and, as a result, can be expected to make greater gains in rehabilitation and respond better to their physical injuries. Conversely, athletes who have negative expectations or engage in negative appraisals of themselves, their situation, or their ability to cope with the ramifications of an injury are less likely to comply with treatment. This cognitive style not only leads to a diminished level of adherence, but it can also have direct and indirect influences on an athlete's subsequent physical recovery. It is important for athletes, their health care team, families, friends, and coaches to evaluate whether the athlete's thoughts and perceptions of their injury and subsequent rehabilitation are contributing to a positive or negative outcome.

Social support within an athlete's personal life as well as their athletic and rehabilitation environments also appears to be an important factor in the injury recovery process. Members of the athletic organization as well as an athlete's friends and partners can play a role in promoting recovery following injury, perhaps by helping them to relieve stress. Psychology professionals and health care providers can certainly function in this capacity as well. Through consultation services or direct treatment provision, members of these professions can provide an invaluable service to individuals as well as athletic organizations. Ultimately, an athlete's response to injury and their subsequent recovery is a multifaceted process. However, working with a knowledgeable and well-informed support staff or a sports medicine team populated by health care professionals from varying disciplines can assist athletes in making sense of their current situation, developing more effective ways of coping, and approaching their physical rehabilitation with a true sense of purpose.

RECOMMENDED READING

Brewer, B., Van Raalte, J. L., Cornelius, A. E., Petitpas, A. J., Sklar, J. H., Pohlman, M. H., Krushell, R. J., & Ditmar, T. D. (2000). Psychological factors, rehabilitation adherence, and rehabilitation outcome following anterior cruciate ligament reconstruction. *Rehabilitation Psychology, 45*, 20–37.

Green, S. L., & Weinberg, R. S. (2001). Relationships among athletic identity, coping skills, social support, and the psychological impact of injury in recreational participants. *Journal of Applied Sport Psychology, 13,* 40–59.

Hanton S., Evans, L., & Neil, R. (2003). Hardiness and the competitive trait anxiety response. *Anxiety, Stress, and Coping, 16,* 167–184.

Harris, L. L. (2003). Integrating and analyzing psychosocial and stage theories to challenge the development of the injured collegiate athlete. *Journal of Athletic Training, 38*(1), 75–82.

Hootman, J. M., Dick, R., & Agel, J. (2007). Epidemiology of collegiate injuries for 15 sports: Summary and recommendations for injury prevention initiatives. *Journal of Athletic Training, 42*(2), 311–319.

Malinauskas, R. (2008). College athletes' perceptions of social support provided by their coach before injury and after it. *Journal of Sports Medicine and Physical Fitness, 48*(1), 107–112.

Sullivan, M. J., Tripp, D. A., Rodgers, W. M., & Stanish, W. (2000). Catastrophizing and pain perception in sport participants. *Journal of Applied Sport Psychology, 12,* 151–167.

Walker, N., Thatcher, J., Lavallee, D. (2007). Psychological responses to injury in competitive sport: a critical review. *Journal of the Royal Society for the Promotion of Health, 127*(4), 174–180.

REFERENCES

Brewer, B. W. (2001). Psychology of sport injury rehabilitation. In Singer, R. N., Hausenblas, H. A., & Janelle, C. M. (Eds.), *Handbook of sport psychology* (2nd ed., pp. 787–809). New York: John Wiley & Sons, Inc.

Brewer, B. W., & Petrie, T. A. (2002). Psychopathology in sport and exercise. In Van Raalte, J. L., & Brewer, B. W. (Eds.), *Exploring sport and exercise psychology* (2nd ed., pp. 307–323). Washington, DC: American Psychological Association.

Gould, D., Udry, E., Bridges, D., & Beck, L. (1997). Coping with season-ending injuries. *Sport Psychologist, 11,* 379–399.

Granito, V. (2002). Psychological response to athletic injury: Gender differences. *Journal of Sport Behavior, 25*(3), 243–259.

Knowles, S. B., Marshall, S. W., Bowling, J. M., Loomis, D., Millikan, R., Yang, J., et al. (2006). A prospective study of injury incidence among North Carolina high school athletes. *American Journal of Epidemiology, 164*(12), 1209–1221.

Kubler-Ross, E. (1969). *On death and dying.* New York: Macmillan.

Newcomer, R. R., & Perna, F. M. (2003). Features of posttraumatic stress disorder among adolescent athletes. *Journal of Athletic Training, 38*(2), 163–166.

Wiese-Bjornstal, D. M., Smith, A. M., Shaffer, S. M., & Morrey, M. A. (1998). An integrated model of response to sport injury: Psychological and sociological dimensions. *Journal of Applied Sport Psychology, 10,* 46–69.

Chapter 7

The Psychological Building Blocks of Exercise, Health, and Fitness: Observations Borne of Experience

Bruce Burke and Kym Burke

By way of introduction, it is important to distinguish among three key terms: exercise, health, and fitness. According to the *American Heritage Dictionary,* exercise is defined as "bodily exertion for the sake of developing or maintaining physical fitness." Scientific studies repeatedly show that staying physically active and exercising regularly can help prevent or delay many diseases and disabilities. Health is defined as "the condition of being sound in body, mind, or spirit; especially: freedom from physical disease or pain." Fitness, on the other hand, is defined as "the state or condition of being fit." For the purposes of this chapter, we would like to extend this definition of fitness to include: *having the physical ability to do what you reasonably may want to for the rest of your life.* It is important to recognize the differences among these key terms. A healthy individual is considered to be free from disease, but may not be necessarily fit. A fit individual is not only healthy (free from disease), but has the aerobic capacity, muscular strength/power, and joint range of motion to permit them to participate in life as they choose. Exercising for health is different from exercising for fitness. Exercising for general fitness is different from exercising for competitive sport.

Individuals approach fitness and exercise from a variety of different perspectives. Some are elite-level athletes, some are baby boomers wanting to get in shape, while others are in their later years of life and simply wish to maintain an active lifestyle. As one personal fitness client so eloquently said, "Hey, I'm not training for the Olympics." While he was not training for competitive sport, the elite athlete indeed *might* need to be reminded that they are, in fact, training for the Olympics. For them, the intensity and focus must always be "on." There is no gray area. Fitness is not so difficult for this person. It is basically a by-product of the way they live their lives. They have the tools, the time, and the financial incentive to do what it takes to succeed.

Most elite athletes have access to all the resources necessary to attain the highest level of fitness. For the rest of the population, fitness may not come as easily. For example, why is it that 60 percent of American adults do not exercise regularly? The benefits of regular exercise have been well documented:

- Reduced risk of heart disease, high blood pressure, osteoporosis, diabetes and obesity
- Increased joint range of motion
- Compressed morbidity
- Enhanced mental health
- Stress and anxiety relief
- Increased energy and stamina
- Improved sleep
- Boosts metabolism
- Burns calories

The paramount question then becomes: If exercise is beneficial for all ages and performance goals, why do so many find it difficult to get started and continue on a program? Why do they find it difficult to overcome inertia and maintain the necessary momentum to receive the benefits of being fit? After all, from a rational standpoint, a program of exercise and proper nutrition can hardly be described as too much to ask for, particularly when an individual's quality of life is in play.

The focus of this chapter is dedicated to identifying the challenges, as well as the solutions for becoming fit. Throughout the chapter, we will draw on our experiences of working with a broad range of clients and occasionally insert actual case studies in order to reinforce our points. As we move forward, we ask: Why have so many "failed" at exercise? What are the keys to a successful exercise experience? What does it mean to be healthy? What does it take to be fit?

Obviously, these are complicated questions, with no single "right" answer for any of them. However, what we do know is that *having the right mindset is almost always a prerequisite to long term success.*

WHY PEOPLE DO NOT EXERCISE
Fear, Self-esteem, and Self-efficacy

Fear of exercise, or rather the exercise experience, has prevented many individuals from even beginning their journey to better health and fitness. Whether it's a fear of failure, a fear of getting hurt, or a fear of looking foolish in front of others, many individuals resign themselves to not being a "workout person." Our society places a premium on appearances. Consequently, for many it's not so much about what they do, but how they look when they are doing it. The self-imposed pressure to conform and perform, especially in the typical health club, is enormous. An individual with a low self-esteem and lack of self-efficacy will find it very difficult to initiate an exercise program. These are the people who believe that they must "get in shape" before joining a fitness facility.

Self-esteem, in terms of having a stable sense of personal worth, affects one's decision-making process in most endeavors, and exercise is no exception. Those individuals possessing high self-esteem not only believe they can cope with the challenges of an exercise regime, they also believe they are *worthy* of the benefits. On the other hand, those whose self-esteem has been damaged, especially in the area of fitness (i.e., previous exercise experience, gym class, etc.), will find it extremely difficult to initiate an exercise program. In addition, there are those whose lifestyle choices have led to poor health and consequently do not feel worthy of the benefits that come from exercise. They believe they deserve what they've got—poor health, disability, etc.

Self-efficacy is defined as "one's belief in one's ability to succeed in specific situations." Self-efficacy plays a central role in the cognitive regulation of motivation because people regulate the level and the distribution of the effort they will expend in accordance with the effects they are expecting. In other words, they put in as much as they think they will get out. If a person believes that exercise will make them feel better and live longer, he or she will work hard at it. If they are not convinced, or even skeptical of the outcome, they will not work hard.

The concept of self-efficacy is the focal point of Albert Bandura's social cognitive theory. According to Bandura, "mastery experience" is the most important factor deciding a person's self-efficacy. Put simply, success raises self-efficacy and failure lowers it. As exercise and fitness often challenges participants to push beyond their comfort zone, it is imperative that the teacher, coach, or trainer set the participant up for success. It is their job to design an effective program and establish a foundation with the participant so they know exactly what is expected. This will prevent the participant from developing unrealistic expectations. It makes little sense for an athlete to believe that he or she can bench press 215 pounds when they have yet to lift 150 pounds. Similarly, a novice runner will need to master 5K runs before they can run a marathon.

Although not as influential as past experience, modeling is a powerful influence when an individual is particularly unsure of him or herself. When people see someone they identify with success, their self-efficacy will increase; and where they see people failing, their self-efficacy will decrease. This is especially powerful if the person being observed appears to have similar abilities and/or limitations. For example, the average person cannot relate to what the media presents as fitness. Media portrayals of well-conditioned models demonstrating exercises serve only to drive the ordinary individual further away. The unfit individual simply cannot see him or herself doing what the fit individual can do.

Finally, a person's perception of their ability to reach a goal can either be increased by positive words of encouragement or decreased by negative words of discouragement. Words of encouragement from a parent or physical education teacher early in a child's life is often all that is needed to give them the confidence to begin and continue an exercise program. Conversely, harsh, critical words spoken to a young person regarding their lack of physical prowess plants seeds of disbelief.

Fear, although often irrational, is another very real roadblock to becoming fit. It is important for the fitness professional to help identify the root of the fear and work with the client accordingly. How does one set the overweight, deconditioned woman with low self-esteem up for success? It certainly is not by talking about the weight issue constantly or spending a lot of time in front of a mirror as they exercise. What about the former star high school football player who has spent the last 30 years building a successful business and is totally out of shape? His fear is that he will look wimpy and might not be able to do something he is asked to do. Many individuals would rather suffer a lifetime of poor fitness and health problems than take a chance on having their ego bruised.

Case Study: Carl—Age 41 (Fear, Self-esteem, Self-efficacy)

Carl had never been much of an athlete, but he always managed to keep himself in decent shape. The last few years were different. Work and family life had begun monopolizing his time. Whatever exercise he once had built into his weekly schedule had disappeared. Inactivity had taken its toll. His body was beginning to ache from poor posture and, mentally, he was battling mild depression. He felt pretty low. It took a lot of courage for him to place the phone call asking for help.

For the first six months of Carl's program, he would walk in the door of our facility with his head down, avoiding eye contact, hoping not to be noticed. As he came out of the locker room, his trainer was right there to greet him and escort him to a "quiet" corner of the gym. After checking in to see how Carl made out after his previous session, his trainer would share the plan for his training session. There were usually very minor "tweaks" to what they had done last time—no surprises. It was extremely important that Carl be successful from session to session, from exercise to exercise, from repetition to repetition. Carl's trainer wisely chose to keep his programming simple but challenging.

In six months, Carl rarely missed a session, As a result, he was becoming genuinely fit and, in his words, "felt better than I did when I was a much younger man." Most importantly, Carl began to regain his self-esteem. He acknowledged that it felt great to be fit again and he was pleased with his effort. He worked it because he knew he was worth it!

Over time, Carl developed trust in his trainer. They began to expand to new, more dynamic exercises. Carl always rose to the challenge. Consequently, Carl began to believe in his ability to accomplish any fitness goal he and his trainer set.

Today Carl lives with the freedom that comes with knowing he is worthy of the goodness that comes with being fit and believes he can physically do anything he sets his mind to.

VISION AND STRATEGY

When Dominique Arnold (a client) set the new American record time in the 110-meter hurdles, he was not surprised. "This is what I've been training for. This is why I do what I do."

How many Olympic athletes have uttered similar words? They have dreamed about the day they would be standing on the podium having the gold medal placed around their necks. That gold medal not only signifies their dominance on the day of competition, but also their unwavering, steadfast commitment to getting results.

Most people can visualize their own "gold-medal" performance. For some, it might be crossing the finish line in the Boston Marathon. For others, it might be reeling in a big fish well into their senior years, or simply maintaining their independence (i.e., being able to put on their socks). So what is the difference between the Olympic athlete and average Joe or Jane exerciser? The answer lies in having a vision then implementing a strategy to make it a reality.

Simply put, vision provides restraint. If we do not have a crystal clear picture of what we want for our health and fitness, we will find it very difficult to be disciplined and self-controlled.

Having a vision is not to be confused with having a goal. Goals have end dates. Goals must be set in accordance with the vision. For example, the woman who sees herself 30 pounds lighter dancing effortlessly at her daughter's wedding might set a goal of exercising 5 days per week and eating nutritiously. Then, as "life" gets in the way and she encounters some roadblocks, her winning strategy will be challenged. The question will then become whether her vision is clear and powerful enough for her to make the right choices.

Successful people focus on the choices they make. Unsuccessful people focus on their circumstances. Without a clear vision and well-thought-out strategy, it is easy to become a victim of our circumstances. It is all too easy to let the many responsibilities that accompany our lives, such as work and family, interfere with becoming fit. Ironically, it is often only a matter of time before the opposite is true—that being unfit interferes with the responsibilities of work and family!

One final word on vision and strategy: It is worth mentioning again—vision provides restraint. A powerful, clear vision will help individuals become disciplined and take responsibility for their circumstances. A lack of discipline should not be confused with laziness. There are many extremely productive individuals that have floundered with their exercise programs not because they are lazy, but because they did not have the vision. They have achieved in other areas of their lives precisely because they were able to envision themselves as productive and successful in those areas.

Elite athletes live by their vision. They never take their eye off their prize. They may not be especially "gifted" with discipline. They simply have a vision. Those of use who are not elite athletes need to ask: How do I see myself today? What do I want to look like? How do I want to feel?

Case Study: Karen (Vision, Strategy)

Thirty-eight-year-old Karen came to our training facility hoping to get some help with her 13-year-old daughter and 11-year-old son. According to Karen, they both needed athletic readiness training. Once we had a strategy in place for her children, as almost a second thought, Karen asked about programming for herself, but had once been a competitive runner, but had obviously let herself go. She was pretty sure she knew what she needed to do, but thought it might be a good idea to get started with a trainer.

During her initial consultation, Karen made sure we had all the right medical information to keep her safe with her training, but was very vague about her goals. Not once did she mention weight loss. I suppose she felt it was unnecessary to state the obvious. We spent the majority of our consultation time discussing the schedule and logistics.

One day, as she was finishing up her training session, she asked her trainer if she had a few moments to talk. The strain in her face and the desperation in her voice were apparent. After a month of training, nothing had changed. It became obvious we had to get to the real issues that were keeping this woman weighed down.

Behind closed doors, Karen began to open up. She shared her extreme disappointment in herself. She was 70–80 pounds heavier than when she retired from the military a few years earlier. She was once a nationally ranked high school cross-country athlete. How could this have happened? "What kind of example am I for my children, especially my daughter?"

It was not like she was not trying. Every morning she would wake up resolved to do things differently. She would make a healthy breakfast for herself, her husband, and the two kids. She would kiss her husband goodbye as he headed out the door and get the kids on the school bus. Before settling into her home office, she would clean up the breakfast dishes, usually nibbling on whatever the kids left behind. Then the negative self-talk would begin. You didn't need to eat that. You just had breakfast. You're not going to lose any weight that way and, "You deserve to be chubby eating that way." The day went pretty much downhill from there.

This woman was hurting. A new approach was needed. We asked if Karen could see herself looking the way she wanted to look. Could she see herself being the wife she wanted to be? Could she see herself being an honorable mother? Could she see herself having a healthy, fit body? She answered "yes" to each question.

Bingo! Once her prize was identified, once she could clearly see the vision, Karen suddenly had the discipline to do what she needed to do nutritionally to support her exercise efforts.

To date, Karen has lost 70 pounds. When asked if she is the woman in her vision, she replied, "Almost." Karen is never going back. As long as she keeps her eye on the prize, she will have the healthy, fit body of her youth.

Case Study: Tina—Age 36 (Vision, Strategy)

It was the summer of 2008. Tina was looking forward to a nice family vacation with her son. Little did she know the terrifying sequence of events that would eventually lead her to take charge of her health and fitness.

Tina was about 100 pounds overweight. Keeping up with little Danny had become quite a challenge. It was easy when he was a baby, but now that he was 6 years old, life had become much more strenuous. Just getting through the activities of daily living usually required a nap in the afternoon. She had become so unfit that she actually described herself as "handicapped."

Tina planned a week at the beach. At the first sight of the ocean, Danny was overtaken with excitement. He took off running, totally disregarding his mother's instructions to stop. Tina was helpless. He was up to his waist before she could even put the beach chair down. Fortunately, the lifeguard spotted the young boy before he got pulled under.

It was at that moment Tina realized that her debilitating obesity was not as much about her anymore as it was about her son. She could not continue living the way she had been living. Doing so would have been the pinnacle of selfishness. Her son deserved better.

She knew she had to lose weight. She had to start eating right and exercising. How was she going to find the motivation on a daily basis to make the right choices? All she needed to do was look at her beautiful little boy. Her vision was to be a healthy, fit mother and role model for her child.

Tina has pictures of Danny on the refrigerator. Her trainer taped a photograph of Danny to the inside cover of her chart. If she ever questioned her next move, she needed only to look at the photos to be reminded why she does what she does and what her vision is.

Tina had a couple of "gold-medal" performances she was training for. One was to be fit enough to take Danny to the zoo. The other was to return to the beach and play in the waves with her son. These "goals" helped to make the vision a reality. She has recently accomplished both.

GENERATIONAL ISSUES

We are "products" of both of our parents. Genetics and heredity have a significant bearing on our lives—in both desirable and undesirable ways. Active parents raise active children. Active children mature into active adults, and the cycle continues. Unfortunately, the opposite is also true; inactive parents raise inactive children. Inactive children mature into inactive adults and, unfortunately, this cycle also continues.

Overcoming generational issues begins with the individual identifying undesirable characteristics and making a *conscious decision* to fight for change. These generational characteristics need to be addressed head-on in order to be successful.

Case Study: Ned—Age 10 (Generational Issues)

A 35-year-old mother of three entered the fitness facility with her overweight 10-year-old son. It was actually the little boy's idea. While out on the playground, he noticed a classmate eagerly playing with the other boys. Fortunately, this young man had the courage to approach the energetic classmate and talk with him. He discovered that the active boy's parent's owned a fitness facility. The obese 10-year-old went right home and told his mom to take him to the fitness facility to get him signed up!

As it turned out, that young man did the work for his whole family. It did not take long for the inactive, deconditioned mom to begin her exercise program with the overweight father right behind. The whole family has been training consistently for the last 9 years.

Case Study: Dotty—Age 76 (Generational Issues)

Dotty has exercised her whole life. Her activities of daily living are such that she needs to be fit truly. She participates in a formal exercise program as a means to ensure her ability to keep up her active lifestyle.

Dotty's 47-year-old daughter, Lori, noticed the positive effects her mom's exercise program was having on her. Although extremely active, Lori had never done any formal exercise; she never felt she needed to. But things were beginning to change. She did not have the energy she used to have. Excess weight was sneaking its way onto her small frame. Formal exercise was clearly working for her mother, so she tried it. She currently trains 3 days a week without fail and feels better than she ever has.

Her 14-year-old son, Billy, participates in sports year-round and is extremely healthy. Through the exposure to formal exercise that his mother and grandmother have provided, he has now decided to start training himself—and he's loving it!

LACK OF EDUCATION

Although becoming fit is not intellectually complicated, the number of myths and outdated protocols that persist is astounding. Many individuals either do not know where to begin or (worse) think they know when they really do not. Beginning an exercise program with limited information will (at best) lead to mediocre results or (at worst) cause injury. Neither is a prescription for long-term success. Indeed, many individuals do not exercise simply because they have not seen any benefit from their exercising in the past. Why exercise if there are no results?

The flip side of having a lack of education is the fact that Americans are constantly being bombarded with too much information through the media. Health clubs, abdominizers, lowfat, low carb, how are they to wade through this deluge of information? Fitness is a $17.6 billion business with many competing theories, approaches, and business practices. In order to sort out the good from the bad, the real from the hype, each individual must carefully determine his or her goals and objectives based on what *they* want, not what Madison Avenue would like them to believe. In order to be successful navigating through this information (and disinformation), one must determine *exactly what their goals and objectives are*. This will allow the individual to concentrate his or her educational efforts in the right direction.

Case Study: Liz—Age 59 (Lack of Education)

Liz is blessed with good genetics. She has always been healthy and looks great. However, she was smart enough to know that she should not take this good health for granted and decided to join a health club. Additionally, she had put on about 10 pounds and wanted to lose them.

The club she joined was 30 minutes away. They told her that she should work out 3 times a week. She is a disciplined individual and wanted to lose the weight, so she made the drive 3 times a week for an entire year. Each time she went in, she did exactly as they told her. Thirty minutes on the treadmill, then go through the circuit of machines. After a full year, she felt a little stronger, but had not lost a pound. It was quite discouraging.

Liz was a perfect candidate to get excellent results from her exercise; she has the discipline! She has a vision and knows where she wants to be. She just needed to be *educated*.

We began by setting her up on a home program so she did not waste 3 hours a week driving. She spent about $100 on some basic equipment, and we spent 5 hours showing her exactly what she needs to do. We educated her on the importance of progression, intensity, variety, and frequency. She now trains herself at home and loves it! She contacts us when she has questions and we meet for update sessions every few months so she can learn some new progressions and exercises.

She is losing the weight and feels better than she has in years. All she needed was the know-how!

PRE-EXISTING MEDICAL ISSUES

Out of the thousands of people we have worked with, 95 pecent of them have preexisting medical issues. Congenital defects, chronic illness, musculoskeletal injuries (acute and overuse) are real issues that must be worked around. Unfortunately, many individuals use their condition as a reason not to exercise at all. A bad knee or back should not be a roadblock to exercise. Poor fitness leads to poor health. That bad knee leads to becoming overweight, which leads to hypertension or worse. The reality is that, with the help of a professional, preexisting conditions can often be helped or eliminated by maintaining an intelligent fitness program. The answer is to focus on what *can* be done, not what cannot.

Case Study: John—Age 65 (Preexisting Medical Condition)

John's back pain reached the point that he could no longer get through a full day's work. He was at the end of his rope. He thought he had tried everything. He had been to a chiropractor, a massage therapist, and a physical therapist, and now he found himself meeting with a surgeon. According to the doctor, John definitely needed to have his back surgically repaired. John was desperate to be rid of the pain. He agreed to have the surgery. What else was he going to do?

The surgery seemed to be a success. He immediately began his postsurgical physical therapy. He never missed a session and was very compliant with his home program. The doctor expected John to be free from pain and capable of doing whatever he wanted as long as he was cautious.

Unfortunately, that is not exactly how things worked out. At the six-month mark, John was noticing that he still struggled to walk without a noticeable limp and still had pain. After returning to the doctor, it was discovered that they had "nicked" a nerve in his back, which was why the muscles of his lower leg were not working properly. As far as the pain, the doctor had no answer.

John did a little research and learned that the first 12 months after surgery were the most critical. Whatever re-education of movement patterns needed to happen, it had to occur in the first 12 months post surgery. John was not about to walk with a limp or be a victim of back pain for the rest of his life. Once again, John found himself desperate but not quite sure where to turn.

Fortunately, he had heard about the work being done by the movement specialists at our fitness facility. After John's initial assessment, a program was designed focusing on the pillars of human movement: pushing, pulling, rotation, and the raising and lowering of our center of gravity and locomotion. (i.e., move across the floor). The training staff chose exercises mimicking these movement patterns. They did not care if John could not do a leg press. They wanted to make sure John could get up and down out of a chair pain free. John trusted his trainers and appreciated the effort put into designing every session. It always amazed him how someone as "fragile" as he was could get such an incredible workout.

To date, John's back pain is under control. "If I didn't do this 'stuff,' I know I'd be right back where I once was." He still has a bit of a "giddy-up" in his step, but it is significantly better than it was. The average person probably would not even notice it.

John is no longer a victim of his back pain. He refuses to focus on what he cannot do, instead choosing to enjoy all that he *is* doing.

TIME

"I don't have the time to exercise." Of all the excuses that we have heard over the years, this is the most common, and probably the worst. When individuals examine their lives honestly, they will almost always come to the realization that they indeed have time to exercise.

As owners of a personal fitness training business, we have had the privilege of being involved in the lives of some very busy, successful people. Whether they have to train at 5:30 in the morning or 8:00 at night, they *always* make time to keep themselves fit. In fact, we think this is what made them successful in the first place—an ability to prioritize and put "first things first."

Think about it—many of the people who "don't have time" to exercise have plenty of time for mowing the lawn, reading a book, working in the garden, taking a nap, whatever. There is certainly nothing wrong with these activities, but these individuals have placed a higher priority on them than on becoming fit. At some point, these people will come to the realization that there is a price to pay for neglecting their fitness. There is no substitute for regular exercise. Indeed, one of the many reasons that people *should* be exercising is so they can stay fit enough to work in the garden until they are 100 years old!

The "no time" issue is quickly placed into perspective by the frequency with which we have observed a person's busy schedule "free up" after they have had a serious medical problem occur in their lives. One cardiac event and they suddenly have all the time in the world to do whatever they must to be healthy. *This happens all the time.* Why not be proactive and work our schedule out so as to prevent this type of life-altering occurrence from happening in the first place? Not only are we taking some preventative medicine, *but we will truly feel better and enjoy our lives more in the process.*

MICROWAVE MENTALITY

American culture has developed in such a way that we have become accustomed to being able to get what we want, when we want it. Perseverance and delayed gratification are long-lost virtues. When it comes to exercising for the sake of fitness, perseverance and delayed gratification are paramount. Determination and resiliency, not entitlement, will lead to success.

Unfortunately, the fitness business and media has preyed on those who are desperate for weight loss, weight gain, six-pack abs, energy of a youngster, etc. Promises of quick results with limited effort are far and wide. It is time to carefully evaluate the facts. The old adage holds true: If it sounds too good to be true, it probably is. There is no fooling the human body. Nobody gets out of shape in one day. Nobody is going to get into shape in one day.

Case Study: Deanna—Age 51 (Microwave Mentality)

It was decided—this was the summer that Deanna was going to get in shape. As a schoolteacher, she found it far too overwhelming to think about adding an exercise program to her already busy schedule.

She had several friends who seemed to be getting great results from their exercise program, so she decided to give it a try. Although she had not exercised regularly for quite some time, she was confident in her ability to jump right in. She did not really think it was necessary to go through an "adaptation phase," as her trainer was suggesting. She just wanted to get ripping!

In the first 14 days of her program, Deanna had exercised 10 times. This was not exactly easing into it. But, in her mind, she did not have a lot of time. This "project" had to be completed by the end of the summer.

After three weeks and very minimal weight loss, Deanna was getting discouraged. She could not understand how she could be working so hard, but seeing so little change in her body composition.

What Deanna came to understand is that decades of inactivity cannot be reversed in three weeks. Although she "felt" like she was working really hard, the reality was that she was not getting that much work done. Her low fitness level was preventing her from performing enough "work" to start tipping the calories in versus calories out in the right direction. It is not unusual to have nonexercisers be out of touch with their fitness reality. Often, it is not until they start exercising that they begin to realize how very out of shape they are.

Deanna trusted our advice and has continued to do as we have asked. She has become progressively more fit and has lost that weight! She has even found time to train during the school year! Funny how time can free up, isn't it?

PREVIOUS EXERCISE EXPERIENCE

Physical Education teachers, coaches, fitness professionals—any and all individuals given the authority to teach physical activity possess a tremendous responsibility for forming the thought patterns associated with exercise. Typically, we make a decision about whether something is "good" or "bad" based on how we feel about it. Emotions often drive our decision-making process. If individuals feel good about themselves as they exercise, they are more likely to repeat the pattern.

Much damage is done in the formative years by insensitive gym teachers, unreasonable coaches, or so-called fitness professionals. For those instructing physical activity, not enough has been done in the area of professional development. Their toolbox might be loaded with exercises, drills, and patterns, but they overlook the most important component—the individual's psyche. Those who are given the authority to lead physical activity must be committed to building the participant up from the inside out.

Case Study: Jan (Fear, Self-esteem, Self-efficacy, Previous Experience)

Forty-nine-year-old Jan was one year away from turning "the Big Five-O." She was in terrible shape and desperately needed to some lose weight. Her old tricks of dieting were not working anymore, and she knew she had to do something to start burning some calories. It took a lot of courage for her to place the phone call, schedule the appointment, and walk through the door of our facility.

At her initial consultation, Jan shared her medical history, goals, and current lifestyle. Fortunately, she was not shy about sharing her extreme distaste for exercise. When questioned further, Jan revealed a couple of childhood memories that had not only affected her self-esteem, but also self-efficacy. A physical education teacher had told her mom that she was hopelessly uncoordinated. Her mom worked with her at home trying to develop the basic motor skills of running, jumping, and throwing. Eventually, she gave up. "Jan, you're never going to be able to throw a ball!" Jan's self-image was that of a pudgy, uncoordinated little girl. She was hopeless until she heard about others in her community experiencing success exercising with a professional personal trainer.

The first training session was critical to the success of Jan's program. We were judicious in her exercise selection. Although challenging, Jan could perform all the exercises her trainer asked her to do. Also, it appeared there was no one else in the gym while they were training. The trainer had Jan so engrossed in what they were doing, she became unaware of the other clients.

Ten years later, Jan is still exercising. She is in excellent health and is able to play ball with her grandchildren.

GETTING STARTED: THE KEYS TO SUCCESS

On August, 11, 2008, I started my exercise program and began eating right. Since then, I have lost 46 pounds, many inches, four sizes in clothing, and lowered both my blood pressure and cholesterol. I am much stronger and both my physical appearance and mental attitude have improved dramatically. I accomplished much more than I ever expected in a short period of time. I feel wonderful! This experience has truly changed my life.

—Nancy D.

Originally, I was happy to just get through a session. Now, it is totally different. I actually look forward to my sessions. I have lost over 50 pounds and feel great! Getting these kinds of results has really motivated me. This exercise program has impacted my quality of life more than I ever could have imagined.

—Ed R.

I am physically capable of enjoying whatever I choose to do. I don't necessarily want to live longer—I want to live well while I'm living. Quality of life is the goal.

—Glenn F.

For these individuals, their commitment to becoming fit has been a life-changing experience. Each person who wants to get fit needs to ask him or herself: What would I be willing to do in order to have a "life-changing" experience? How much time could I set aside in my busy schedule to be physically capable of enjoying whatever I choose to do as I age? Of course, this all sounds *really, really* good. So how does one get started? How does one ensure success?

To begin with, there is no "one-size-fits-all" solution. Different individuals have different physical limitations and goals. As each individual charts their course, it is important to differentiate between exercise for exercise sake and incidental exercise. Many experts extol the virtues of walking 20 minutes a day or taking the stairs instead of the elevator. While these are both great ideas and significantly better than doing nothing, your *fitness* goals aren't going to be realized by simply walking and taking the stairs.

There is a reasonable school of thought that believes that any type of low-intensity movement is better than nothing at all, particularly for the general population. There is no question that this is true. In addition, everyone knows how to walk and climb stairs, so it is a pretty safe recommendation that is readily available. It is relaxing, you can do it with your friends, and it costs nothing. Most importantly, *it will absolutely have a positive impact on your health.* At a glance, it seems like the perfect exercise regimen. However, such rudimentary exercise will not allow you to become truly fit. It will not, by itself, allow you to physically do whatever you reasonably like for the rest of your life.

A walking program can be a great solution to the "too much information" problem. If the objective is to do something modest to impact health without having to think about it too much, a walking program is quite possibly the answer. If becoming truly fit as we have described it is the goal, a more comprehensive approach is required. As always, start with a vision, then create goals, objectives, and a strategy to attain them.

INTELLIGENT EXERCISE

The American College of Sports Medicine (ACSM) and the American Heart Association (AHA) updated their exercise guidelines in 2007 for the first time in 12 years. Here are the updated guidelines:

For healthy adults under age 65:

- Do moderately intense cardio 30 minutes a day, five days a week, or vigorously intense cardio 20 minutes a day, 3 days a week; and
- Do eight to 10 strength-training exercises, 8 to 12 repetitions of each exercise twice a week.

Moderate-intensity physical activity means working hard enough to raise your heart rate and break a sweat, yet still being able to carry on a conversation. It should be noted that to lose weight or maintain weight loss, 60 to 90 minutes of physical activity may be necessary. The 30-minute recommendation is for the average healthy adult to maintain health and reduce the risk for chronic disease.

For adults over 65:

- Do moderately intense aerobic exercise 30 minutes a day, five days a week, or vigorously intense aerobic exercise 20 minutes a day, 3 days a week; and
- Do 8 to 10 strength-training exercises, 10 to 15 repetitions of each exercise twice to three times per week; and
- If you are at risk of falling, perform balance exercises; and
- Have a physical activity plan.

Both aerobic and muscle-strengthening activity is critical for healthy aging. Moderate-intensity aerobic exercise means working hard at about a level-6 intensity on a scale of 1–10. You should still be able to carry on a conversation during exercise. In addition, older adults or adults with chronic conditions should develop an activity plan with a health professional to manage risks and take therapeutic needs into account. This will maximize the benefits of physical activity and ensure your safety.

As noted, these guidelines were updated in 2007 for the first time since 1995. For the general population, it is difficult to keep up with the latest recommendations, protocols, and techniques. Many may still firmly believe that the 1995 guidelines are "gospel." Those who are looking for kinder, softer recommendations should continue to believe so. The reality is that the new recommendations are asking for more from each individual, regardless of age.

The ACSM and AHA listed several "improvements" to the new guidelines including;

Moderate-intensity physical activity has been clarified.

The 1995 document simply specified "most, preferably all days per week" as the recommended frequency, while the new recommendation identifies 5 days per week as the recommended.

Vigorous-intensity physical activity has been explicitly incorporated into the recommendation.

To acknowledge both the preferences of some adults for vigorous-intensity physical activity and the substantial science base related to participation in such activity, the recommendation has been clarified to encourage participation in moderate- and/or vigorous-intensity physical activity. Vigorous-intensity physical activity was implicit in the 1995 recommendation. It is now explicitly an integral part of the physical activity recommendation.

Specified: Aerobic activity needed is in addition to routine activities of daily life.

The updated recommendation now clearly states that the recommended amount of aerobic activity (whether of moderate or vigorous intensity) is in addition to routine activities of daily living which are of light intensity, such as self-care, casual walking, or grocery shopping; or less than 10 minutes of duration, such as walking to the parking lot or taking out the trash. Few activities in contemporary life are conducted routinely at a moderate intensity for at least 10 minutes in duration. However, moderate- or vigorous-intensity activities performed as a part of daily life (e.g., brisk walking to work, gardening with shovel, or carpentry) performed in bouts of 10 minutes or more can be counted towards the recommendation. Although implied, this concept was not effectively communicated in the original recommendation.

"More is better."

The new recommendation emphasizes the important fact that physical activity above the recommended minimum amount provides even greater health benefits. The point of maximum benefit for most health benefits has not been established but likely varies with genetic endowment, age, sex, health status, body composition, and other factors. Exceeding the minimum recommendation further reduces the risk of inactivity-related chronic disease. Although the dose-response relation was acknowledged in the 1995 recommendation, this fact is now explicit.

Muscle-strengthening recommendation is now included.

Muscle-strengthening activities have now been incorporated into the physical activity recommendation. Although the 1995 recommendation mentioned the importance of muscular strength and endurance, it stopped short of making specific declarations in this area. Available evidence now allows the integration of muscle strengthening activities into the core recommendation.

These "improvements" all have a common theme that must be acknowledged: more is better! It has done our nation no good to believe that the bare minimum (which is what the guidelines are) is all that is necessary for us to stay healthy, much less fit. It is a very good start—better than nothing—but that is it. The statistics show that our old strategies have not been working.

DEVELOPING AN INTELLIGENT APPROACH TO FITNESS

It is hard to say what is *the most* important component of a successful, lifelong fitness program, but certainly one of the more important is the individual's *mindset*. We cannot tell you how many times we have seen someone fail who has been really motivated to lose weight and do whatever it takes to get there. Some people start their effort by living a truly unrealistic and unsustainable lifestyle. They work out more than they should and eat significantly less than they should. There is no question they will lose weight doing this, but at what price? They are miserable and ultimately end up right back where they started.

Another approach that does not work consistently is focusing on weight and not fitness. If the goal is simply weight loss, it is easy to become demoralized when it does not happen fast enough. As was mentioned earlier, a "quick fix" mentality can sabotage a realistic effort to attain fitness.

So what does work? When people approach their exercise program from the perspective of simply wanting to become fit and have it be sustainable for the long term, they tend to succeed. Why wouldn't they? They have no unmet expectations and begin to truly appreciate how good "fitness" feels. Having realistic expectations is key.

A concept we strongly believe in is the concept of "living outside your comfort zone." People are a product of their environment and the stimuli that they encounter. Life in their "comfort zone" reflects how they look and feel on a day-to-day basis. If they want to look and feel differently, they have to be willing to live differently. In order to see *extra-ordinary* results, you have to be willing to do *extra-ordinary* things.

A SUCCESSFUL START

Getting off to a good start is critical to the long-term success of a fitness program. Those who develop programs on their own frequently miss this extremely important part of the fitness puzzle. They begin by making a decision to start exercising. Most often it is for the right reason: to become more fit. They then take their limited understanding of what it takes to become fit and "give it a shot." It might be basketball, running, lifting weights, sit-ups, whatever they may have access to or think they know how to do. As always, *success is measured by the attainment of their goals and objectives*. Some people may be successful this way, but how many of them become injured? How many of them are lifting weights and doing sit-ups but are not losing any weight?

There is another group of "do-it-yourselfers" that, unlike the previous group, start their program for the *wrong* reasons. "I have a wedding coming up in two months and need to lose 40 pounds." These individuals usually get involved in quick weight loss schemes that can actually cause more harm than good.

A key component to a successful exercise program involves the individual's personal responsibility and discipline of *owning* their fitness program. Unfortunately, many individuals do not have the tools to set up an appropriate fitness program. Those interested in developing a fitness program on their own should begin by becoming educated about fitness in order to ensure a successful start. We believe that meeting with a true fitness professional, even for a few sessions, provides the best opportunity to do just that.

Case Study: Steve—Age 39 (A Successful Start)

When Steve first came to us, he had never done anything physical in his life. He had joined a health club a few times, but that never worked. His goals were pretty generic. He basically just wanted to get stronger, lose a few pounds, and be fit. He said that as much as anything, he wanted to make it part of his lifestyle. He wanted to be educated, and he wanted to be held accountable.

Steve worked with one of our trainers three days a week for about a year. He was seeing great results, but wanted to see if he would have the discipline to do it on his own. He started meeting with his trainer once per week and trained himself the rest of the time.

Today, Steve is fully independent, checking in with us whenever he needs an update or has a question. He feels better than he ever has and has described his experience as "life changing." He is determined never to go back to the way he was. He is living his vision.

Having a Successful Start Requires:

- Having a clear vision and goals that will help you realize that vision.
- Goals that are realistic and attainable.
- Understanding what is expected and required from the outset.
- Knowing, specifically, what types of exercises and protocols will lead to success.
- Not feeling overwhelmed.
- A conservative approach to exercise frequency and intensity.
- Avoiding injury.
- Maintaining realistic expectations during each session; no bruised ego!
- Finishing each exercise session saying, "That wasn't so bad!"

Initial success will lead to improved confidence, which in turn will lead to increased desire. Deconditioned individuals who begin exercising correctly feel *significantly* better in a relatively short amount of time. Their margin for improvement is markedly higher than that of an already fit person. Implementing an exercise program is not unlike building a house. The foundation must be built first, and it must be built well in order for the rest of the house to be strong. There can be no long-term success without having a strong foundation.

LONG-TERM SUCCESS

Once the house is built, it must be maintained for the long haul. Long-term success requires:

- Consistent exercise frequency.
- Intelligent departures from individual comfort zones; regular exposure to different loads and stimuli.
- Variety. A successful program must be fun!
- Avoiding injury. Consult with an exercise professional regularly.

Commitment leads to positive outcomes. Positive outcomes lead to greater commitment.

IDENTIFYING A FITNESS PROFESSIONAL

The process of identifying a fitness professional is complicated by a lack of national standardization regarding training, experience, and certification. There are many paths to becoming a fitness professional, some better than others. As is the case in many people-oriented professions, "book knowledge" does not necessarily translate into success as a personal trainer. The best advice is to ask for references and use common sense when interviewing personal trainers. Several Internet-based sites may be helpful, including: http://www.acsm.org and http://www.acefitness.org.

If exercise is beneficial for all ages and performance goals, why do so many find it difficult to get started and continue on an exercise program? We hope the information contained in this chapter has shed light on why so many have found it difficult to overcome inertia and/or maintain the momentum necessary to experience success with their exercise programs.

In order to be successful, the individual must identify a prize he or she finds worth pressing for. They have to own it. Once they own it, the commitment will flow from their passion, which in turn will help them drop their destructive habits and mindsets. This then lays the foundation for acquiring new, supportive behaviors and thought patterns.

In conclusion, we encourage you to examine your approach, seek the truth and experience the freedom that comes with being healthy and fit. For most, it becomes life-changing.

AUTHORS' NOTE

This chapter should help the reader identify and navigate through the challenges people face as they consider becoming fit, as well as encourage each individual to strive for and achieve their personal fitness goals. The observations and recommendations come from our personal experience. The case studies are all from clients we have worked with over the years. In most instances, the names have been changed to ensure confidentiality. In the case of testimonials, permission has been granted to post their comments in this chapter.

Chapter 8

Psychological Care of Student-Athletes in a University Environment

Desi Alonzo Vásquez Guerrero, Donna K. Broshek, Jason R. Freeman, and Katherine E. Cutitta

Student-athletes face an array of unique challenges and often present to sports medicine physicians and other professionals seeking various types of assistance ranging from post-injury recovery to academic concerns or personal problems. As the roles of psychologists on sports medicine teams have increased in many university athletic settings, so has the need for expanding the literature guiding the psychological treatment and assessment of student-athletes in the hope of developing more effective evidence-based approaches for therapeutic care. For the psychologist, part and parcel of providing ethical care to athletes is understanding the crucible-like environment of pressures and relationships in which the athletes are expected to perform. Additionally, it is important to be mindful of the developmental tasks and individual factors that impact a student-athlete's health, well-being, and performance. With these issues in mind, this chapter discusses the university environment in which many student-athletes live and work, the developmental factors that mitigate or exacerbate psychopathology, and reviews approaches for assessing and treating student-athletes.

THE ACADEMIC VILLAGE

The university environment is replete with individuals, institutions, organizations, and other stakeholders demanding time and attention from the student-athlete. These entities include coaches and coaching staff, administrators, medical teams, professors and classes, teammates, and classmates. Also, athletes often strive to maintain relational networks of family members and friends back home, or manage romantic relationships that may have recently begun or ended. Just as demanding are the student-athletes' individual desires to succeed and to uphold or improve their school's athletic reputation.

Thus, student-athletes entering the academic village are faced with a stunning array of demands from various entities and the networks of relationships they represent. Using what might be described as Herculean effort, the student-athlete is expected to successfully navigate these relational systems while achieving feats of competitive prowess on the playing field, pursuing an education, and continuing the maturation process into adulthood with some measure of personal fulfillment. Beginning with the coach and coaching staff, a deeper understanding of a student-athlete's relationship with some of these major stakeholders will allow psychologists to better assess the contextual factors that influence a student-athlete's psychological health.

Coaches

Initially, it is often the relationships with the new coach and coaching staff that are given the utmost importance by the student-athlete. The student-athletes were typically recruited to play by these university coaches, who frequently offer the student-athletes financial support. Coaches may have also promised the athlete a starting role, or the possibility of playing for professional or Olympic teams in order to secure a commitment. These rewards are typically conditional on making progress in the sport and the coaches' continued approbation. Thus, the student-athlete may have a tremendous feeling of responsibility to continue pleasing the coach to maintain scholarships and attain these goals.

Student-athletes' families may also demonstrate loyalty to and dependence on the coaches and coaching staff. Student-athletes and their families may realize that the student would not have qualified academically or be financially able to matriculate into the university, especially a selective institution, without athletic ability. For students coming from families with non-collegiate backgrounds, parents and student-athletes may find themselves trusting the coaches to "take care" of the students as they venture away from their parents into the college environment. Additionally, there may be a "handing off" process from a high school or club-level coach to the university-level coach.

Regardless of the actual method by which the student-athlete transfers to the care of the university coaching staff, the student-athlete's perception of loyalty and level of dependence on the coach may magnify the impact of that relationship on the student-athlete when problems arise. For a student-athlete who trusts his or her coach, the coaching relationship may be the first place an athlete mentions a problem, whether academic, athletic, or personal in nature. A supportive coach may also be more likely to notice problems with the student's performance or emotional functioning and may also be more likely to make a referral to either the medical staff or team psychologist. Conversely, student-athletes who have less supportive relationships with their coaches may attempt to conceal or minimize their problems for fear that the head coach may view them as weak or inadequate with a resultant impact on their playing time. These student-athletes may turn to other members of the coaching or medical staff to discuss problems. Regardless, the coaching or medical staffs are frequently the first points of contact for the student-athletes when they need assistance.

Initially, the types of problems presented to coaching or medical staff may take the form of academic, performance, or post-injury recovery issues, but for various reasons, these presenting problems may only be the "tip of the iceberg." The underlying issues or more severe problems may be revealed only as issues are explored in an initial meeting, or perhaps only subsequently with the team psychologist. Student-athletes may frequently employ a "cover issue" if their primary problem is with their coach or teammates, if they perceive their problems to be more serious in nature, or if the problem may be considered taboo by some, such as dealing with sexual orientation.

At this point, the importance of medical staff who emphasize their dedication to student-athletes' health, their openness to all concerns, and their willingness to advocate cannot be overemphasized. Athletic trainers and team physicians form an important part of the referral process to psychologists as well as valuable liaisons. If student-athletes perceive the medical staff or psychologist as an extension of the team, they may feel trapped and unable to receive needed help.

Interestingly, psychologists dealing with multiple players from a team may notice that athletes from the same team appear to deal with similar issues. Some of this may be due to the nature of the sport itself, such as eating disorders in long-distance runners or other athletes such as wrestlers who need to decrease their weight rapidly to make weight classes, issues with coaches, team dynamics, or disciplinary problems. The coach or coaching staff may also inadvertently exacerbate preexisting issues and at times discussions between the psychologist and coaching staff may become necessary, with the student-athlete's permission. Even a coach with the best intentions may become too involved in the student-athletes' personal difficulties and boundaries between the psychology, sports medicine, and coaching staff may need to be established or clarified. Depending on the nature of the problems and the extent of the issues, teamwide interventions may become appropriate.

In conclusion, the university environment houses a variety of entities and relationships demanding a student-athlete's time and attention. Initially, the student-athlete may view the relationship with their coach as the most important of these relationships and as one that can offer a significant amount of support and encouragement to the student-athlete. The coach or coaching staff, however, may also inadvertently exacerbate preexisting or emerging issues, and it is important that members of the sports medicine team, including psychologists, make it clear that their primary responsibility lies in providing ethical care for the student-athlete.

Teammates

Just as coaches set team policy and regulations, they also sow the seeds of team culture by choosing a student-athlete's teammates. It is the older and fellow players who are most likely to teach the unwritten rules, the "dos and don'ts" of a student-athlete's new environment, on and off the court or field. It is also the older teammates who may first accept or ostracize a new player because of their willingness to comply with unwritten rules, or other issues. A younger athlete will therefore likely defer towards older, likely more successful, athletes during practices when it comes to interpreting what the coach is asking for when giving instructions. Through older teammates' reactions to the coaches, the younger athlete may also begin to form impressions of the other players' attitudes to the coaches, to training, or even to what type of behavior is appropriate off the court or off the field. These impressions may include perceptions of the importance of academics in the lives of student-athletes.

Other teammates are also likely to be a significant source of feedback and self esteem for new players regarding their performance and presence on the team. Positive affirmation from older players may boost a younger student-athlete's confidence and encourage greater levels of performance. Harsh or overly critical feedback could have the opposite effect.

One concern sometimes expressed by older players is feeling challenged by younger, possibly more heavily recruited players. This issue may occur more often in older players who have experienced injuries or have not felt like they have reached their athletic potentials. Thus, a highly competitive player or highly competitive incoming class may ruffle the feathers of the members of the older classes, especially if these new players are more quickly promoted to key positions or given leadership responsibilities, and the older players are left feeling passed up or challenged by younger players' athletic abilities, or demonstrated performance. This may result in resentment towards younger players, or it may pique preexisting anxiety or guilt in older players about their own progress on the team and whether they really "have it in them" to succeed. Coaches may intentionally or inadvertently exacerbate some of these tensions if comparisons are made between older players and incoming student-athletes.

Because student-athletes spend so much time with their teammates, they form a very important, and sometimes the only, social group for new student-athletes. Due to scheduling demands, it may be extremely difficult for players to initiate or maintain relationships outside of their teammates, reinforcing the strength of the team's norms and social values. Therefore, norms regarding a student-athlete's disclosure of emotional, psychological, or relational issues to others may be set more by the team culture than by any other social or relational group on campus. Similar to the effect that their relationship with the coaching staff would have, a student-athlete may feel more or less willing to share personal problems with other players, and may feel more or less supported in a decision to seek professional assistance from team psychologists, based on the perceived potential reactions of their teammates. Thus, teammates may exacerbate or mitigate specific issues that the athletes are experiencing. Unsupportive teammates may reduce the likelihood of someone self-disclosing personal difficulties, whereas supportive teammates may be the first to notice problems when they occur and suggest that the student-athlete seek professional guidance.

Psychologists treating student-athletes may find themselves treating multiple players from the same team. From a clinical perspective, this may allow the psychologist to see the inner workings of the team from multiple standpoints, which may be helpful. At the same time, accumulated knowledge of the team's inner workings may also bring the psychologist into enmeshed and entangled relationships among student-athletes or the team itself, and the feeling of being "caught in the middle." From a systems perspective, some student-athletes may also engage in some "splitting" or team sabotage. Issues of confidentiality may also arise when psychologists forget which student-athletes disclosed what facts. Thus, extra care may need to be exercised by the psychologist when treating multiple members of the same athletics team.

In sum, student-athletes' teammates play a considerable role in their lives. This influence can pervade several spheres, including playing time, specific training or other team issues, off-court behavior, and likelihood of professional help-seeking, and may even change the in-room dynamics of therapy sessions when treating multiple athletes from the same team. It is therefore important that team psychologists acknowledge the considerable influence that team members have on a student-athlete, in addition to the influence of coach and coaching staff, and that psychologists be thoughtful about ways to address the ramifications. Lastly, just as new on-campus relationships with coaches and teammates can wield powerful influences over student-athletes, so can the personal relationships at home, namely those with families-of-origin and romantic relationships.

Parents

Students will have varying degrees of support from families-of-origin for both athletic and academic performance, as well as individual health and well-being. The nature of parental support may depend largely on factors such as previous parental involvement, parental socioeconomic status, proximity to the college, and parental level of investment that may or may not depend upon whether the parent was a former athlete or coach. Some parents, especially those who were former athletes themselves or who were previously highly involved in their children's sports, may continue to be involved while their young adult child is competing at the university level. This may be especially true in the case of Olympic sports, where direct family involvement may have been historically more important to a child's success due to the individual nature of the sport. In contrast to non-Olympic sports, like football programs that are typically better funded, many Olympic sports may have diminished funding from high schools or clubs. Parents of exceptional athletes have often made significant sacrifices so that their sons and daughters could continue to have the chance to succeed in these sports, including driving them to nearby towns for practices, sports camps, and otherwise spending significant time and money on training.

Families' socioeconomic resources may also affect student-athletes. For example, athletes from poorer families may sense that some type of university-level stardom or professional success may rescue their family-of-origin from parents' unfulfilled dreams or from financial difficulties. Student-athletes may even be the first members of their families to attend college, or perceive themselves to be one of the few members of their community to "get away from" their hometown. Alternatively, students from high-achieving families may feel responsible for continuing their families' aspirations or accomplishments, and parents may live out their own failed athletic dreams through the accomplishments of their children. In either situation, pressure from parents, perceived and real, may even increase as their child experiences increasing levels of success.

To conclude, students will have varying degrees of support from families-of-origin, which may differentially affect the way that an athlete presents to psychologists or affect the nature of the presenting problems. Thus, it is important for psychologists to review family-of-origin issues with student-athletes early in therapy to gauge ways that family involvement may, or may not be beneficial to their coping.

Romance

As with the relationships previously described, student-athletes' romantic relationships may be sources of both tremendous support and stress for the student-athletes. Student-athletes involved with other student-athletes, regardless of team affiliation, may experience greater levels of understanding from their partners because of the similar time demands and athletic pressures. If the couple is on the same team, they may benefit from being able to spend time together at sporting events, especially when things are going well within the relationship. When things are going poorly between student-athlete couples, however, being on the same athletic team may become a source of extra stress. Student-athletes may feel that they are not getting enough space from each other, or that the team is overly involved, or that both team and individual performance are being hampered by the strain associated with the stressful relationship.

When couples are on different sports teams, then practice, travel, and academic schedules may work to produce a logistical nightmare regarding when student-athletes might be able to spend time together. The same logistical barriers or other misunderstandings may also cause stress when student-athletes date nonathletes. Members of extremely high-profile teams such as men's basketball and football may have added pressures related to doubts regarding their romantic partners' true interests in them and long-term commitment in the relationship. For the psychologist, it often becomes important to guide the athlete in recognizing the strengths and weaknesses in these relationships, and identifying his or her role within them. For serious relational issues, couples counseling for the student-athletes may be indicated, though in cases where there are preexisting individual therapeutic relationships, a specific referral for couples counseling may be appropriate.

Pressures of Standing, Scholarship, and Press

Incredible pressure can be placed on players to live up to the expectations for which they were recruited. Depending on the university's national or regional conference reputation, these pressures may include team expectations that the new student-athlete will revive a dying athletic program, or improve or maintain the team's regional or national standings. Players may seek to surpass these expectations and make sure they are not the "weak link" or the one who "can't cut it." These pressures may also be interwoven with pressures related to scholarship awards. Unfortunately, recent research revealed that male basketball players' receipt of full scholarships was associated with higher internal feelings of pressure, including anxiety and guilt (Medic, Mack, Wilson, & Starkes, 2007). Press coverage of student-athlete performance, on and off the "field" of competition, can exacerbate these feelings of pressure, anxiety, and guilt.

Though there may have been some press coverage of the athletes in hometown newspapers or radio programs, the increased level of public scrutiny and the nature of the coverage at the Division I level may create feelings of living in a "fishbowl." Radio programs and national media attention focus on players and their personal "stories." Student-athletes' stats, athletic histories, academic status, and possibly personal details will be broadcast and discussed via television, radio, the Internet, and print. Spotlighting is likely to increase as athletes gain notoriety, and demonstrate increasing success, failures, or even personal flaws, poor judgment, or legal difficulties.

The nature of the press coverage typically changes once the student-athlete reaches the Division I level of competition. High school student-athletes may have been covered in their local news media for generally positive issues, with any negative attention curtailed by the student's youth or the personal concern that local news media may have for the student and a desire to see them succeed. At the conference or national level, different priorities can result in diminished focus on the individual student-athlete's needs, with greater emphasis given to perceived performance, team performance, role on the team, or perceived potential to enter the professional sports or Olympic-level arenas. Because the student-athletes are adults, the level of press intrusion will increase from that at the high school level, and any personal problems or brushes with the law or other missteps will likely be magnified. Athletes from certain sports will also have the intense pressure of continuing on to national-, Olympic-, and professional-level competitions.

INDIVIDUAL AND DEVELOPMENTAL FACTORS
Biological Factors

Even as student-athletes navigate the pressures of the academic village, it may be difficult to see them as normal students because of the air of confidence they project, the breadth of their achievements, or even their physical presence. It is a mistake, however, to regard student-athletes as "superhuman" or even as "super-healthy" physically or psychologically. Instead, student-athletes are similar to other traditionally aged college students in that they are entering late adolescence and moving into adulthood, which may be a time of emerging biological, physical, or emotional vulnerability. Such vulnerability might include physical problems due to past injury or overtraining, as well as susceptibility to emotional problems, including anxiety and mild depression, or less common psychiatric disorders such as bipolar disorder or psychotic disorders.

In fact, due to rigorous and constant training schedules, student athletes may also be at heightened risk for injuries. As reported by Etzel and Watson (2007), the training environment has changed significantly for university-level athletes over the past 20 years, becoming more complex, more durable, and highly specialized. Even when athletes are officially or technically relieved from training responsibilities due to NCAA regulations, student-athletes are often pressured to participate in "voluntary" training sessions, possibly sponsored by team captains or other team leaders. Student-athletes may face some level of punitive treatment when they decline to participate, or may feel intrinsic pressure to maintain fitness or skill levels.

This unremitting schedule of grueling, all-year training places student-athletes at increasing risk for overtraining, inadequate recovery time, and burnout. While their bodies are continuing to mature and they are dealing with significant stress, student-athletes are also attempting to establish a personal identity, accomplish academic goals, and identify career goals, which may be distinct from those discussed previously with parents, professors, or coaches. In fact, through biological and hormonal processes, overtraining can actually increase risk of injury and significantly lengthen post-recovery periods due to constant levels of increased psychological distress, increased fatigue levels, impaired muscle growth, and a compromised immune system. Similarly, overtraining may also increase the likelihood of psychological distress at a time when adolescents, especially adolescent males, are living through the peak ages of emergence of mental illness. Elevated levels of cortisol, a hormone associated with stress and other measures of psychological distress, have been associated with negative mood states and mood instability.

Identity Issues/Professional Goals

For many athletes at the Division 1 level, their lives have likely revolved around sports since middle school or junior high school. The more elite and more successful the athlete, the more time they have likely spent in training, being immersed in sport team culture, and the greater number of years they have spent participating in the sport. With so much time spent training and competing, much of a student-athlete's identity may revolve around being in sports. As most of the student-athletes being recruited at the Division I level will have been immensely successful, most student-athletes may have found themselves ostensibly comfortable with their identities as athletes.

Once thrown into the university setting, however, student-athletes who have previously been highly regarded and possibly known as the most talented players in their hometowns, or even states, may find themselves to be only average or even a lower-performing team member compared to other new recruits or older teammates. Athletes who once got "a lot of play time" on the court or consistently played in the most strategic positions on the field may find themselves playing for less time, taking on supportive roles, or sometimes not even playing at all. This is often a significant shock to the student-athlete's ego or self-esteem and can cause second-guessing and doubts about self-worth, identity, or future career goals.

While some athletes may be faced with the real possibility of being drafted or competing at a national or international level, others must cope with disappointment and the loss of lifelong dreams. Student-athletes who have expected to advance to professional- or Olympic-level competition may for the first time, and late in their academic careers, realize that these aspirations are not reasonable, possibly causing a major realignment of their identities, feelings toward athletics, and academic or professional goals. Unfortunately, prior academic and professional decisions thus far might have been influenced or made by coaches or coaching staff, or by athletics academic counselors, with a possible conflict of interest. Rather than supporting student-athletes in developing their own academic agenda, athletics personnel may have encouraged them to pursue more flexible or less academically demanding degree requirements in order to maintain rigorous training regimens.

Even within their majors, elite-level athletes may not have excelled to the same degree in school or in other endeavors due to the time demands of their sports, putting them at a disadvantage when compared to other students. Moreover, when players realize that they are not experiencing as much athletic success as they hoped for, they may feel trapped in athletics because they are in a double-bind. For example, some students who have realized that professional-level or Olympic-level competition is unreasonable may wish to redouble their efforts towards academics; however, those energized efforts at academic success may be muted by the continuing demands of athletics. Yet, these same students cannot afford to attend their present institution without an athletic scholarship, which they would most assuredly lose if they quit the team. In these situations, goal clarification and transparent communication by student-athletes with those involved in such decisions are essential components of sessions with a team psychologist.

Some student-athletes in these situations may even attempt to negotiate a life that is separate from athletics in preparation for graduation or other life changes, regardless of athletic or academic success. This may incur losses of friendship, of dreams, of parents' approval, and disillusionment that relationships with others may not have gone deeper than a mutual interest in sports. Some students who do not continue in athletics may also worry about the imminent loss of prestige, privilege, and even self-esteem that accompanied their identity as an athlete at a Division I school.

Student-athletes faced with the realities of separating themselves from athletics, whether due to graduation, academics, or performance reasons, may also feel a sense of confusion or even betrayal and bitterness toward the possibility that they were "used" or "taken advantage of" by the university, with black males being most likely to develop negative feelings toward their academic institutions (Parham, 1993). In short, their sport had truly become a "real" place and setting of their lives, where they ate, had medical care, and lived with other athletes, and then "almost overnight," athletics and the associated benefits and resources are gone.

Moreover, regardless of how student-athletes feel about their participation in athletics or their athletic futures, they are like other late adolescents who are learning how to individuate themselves from their families-of-origin or prior social cultures, attempting to carve out their own lives, identities, and worldviews. Some of the issues that student-athletes may be confronting for the first time, and without direct parent involvement, include broader social issues, such as race, religion, politics, sexual orientation, values, or a host of other topics with which they compare and contrast to their experiences growing up. Because of athletic involvement, wrestling through many of these issues may be delayed or put on hold because the athlete has more pressing demands. Eventually, life events may force these topics into greater importance, either gradually or all at once. Psychologists can be helpful to athletes who may be dealing with some of these issues for the first time in their adult lives.

CLINICAL ISSUES

Impulsivity, Coping Skills, and Risky Behavior

As reviewed above, there is a strong body of evidence that suggests student-athletes in university-level athletics programs are dealing with considerable pressures. Though many of these pressures are similar in nature to those of other students, student-athletes must handle these pressures and developmental tasks in a unique context—juggling two full-time jobs and the accompanying athletic identities and responsibilities. At the same time, student-athletes are not necessarily better equipped to deal with these issues, compared to other students. In fact, research suggests that on average, student-athletes experienced lower levels of well-being on an evidence-based measure of wellness when compared to nonathletes. Student-athletes can experience depression, anxiety, eating disorders, substance abuse, and problems with self-esteem with just as much or greater frequency than the general student population. These issues may be worse for those student-athletes from lower socioeconomic or poorer academic backgrounds.

Performance stress, academic pressures, balancing multiple relationships, and social isolation, coupled with immature coping skills, may increase the likelihood of using ineffective or destructive methods for coping with problems, such as alcohol or substance abuse, or violence. Indeed, student-athletes are more likely to report higher rates of alcohol and substance abuse than nonathletes, more likely to engage in binge drinking, and more likely to suffer negative consequences (e.g., academic problems, criminal behavior, and risky sexual behavior) related to alcohol compared to nonathletes. Team leaders are significantly more likely than teammates to binge drink. Particular team cultures may also contribute to differential rates between teams when alcohol and substance abuse are measured. The same team culture may also affect attitudes toward professional help-seeking for substance abuse issues.

Intervention

As reviewed in Bennet (2007), Broshek & Freeman (2005), and Gardner (2007a), a multidisciplinary, comprehensive, and evidence-based approach to the therapeutic care of athletes is essential to dealing with the broad array of pressures, concerns, and psychological issues that athletes experience during practices and competitions, as well as in their personal lives. In this section, we briefly review exemplars of treatment approaches to treating issues occurring in the competitive athletic setting, as well as more generalized clinical and personal nonclinical concerns before proposing a model of care.

First, as pointed out by others, work with student-athletes can and should include preventative care beginning at the time of recruitment. This can include presentations to recruited student-athletes, their families, coaches, team medical staff, and nutritionists regarding problems often experienced by student-athletes, including psychological disorders, social stressors, adjustment reactions, and risky coping behaviors. These presentations should be aimed at mobilizing resources for recognizing, reducing, and eliminating behavioral risk factors such as suicidal ideation, binge drinking, other substance abuse, and risky sexual behavior. Relationships between possible athletic performance, performance anxiety, and other pressures should be explained, emphasizing the shared goals of optimizing the student-athlete's success and experience in all arenas.

Student-athletes and their families, as well as coaches and medical staff, need to be made aware that late adolescence, especially for men, is a vulnerable time when clinical issues may arise that have not been encountered before or preexisting issues may be exacerbated or triggered by intense physical or mental stress. Lack of social support may also lead to increased vulnerability to psychological problems, whereas the presence of social support may help build resilience. Athletes should also be informed that alcohol and other substance abuse may increase vulnerability to psychological disorders or constitute their etiology. Remedial or disciplinary actions for student-athletes caught breaking team rules or committing other infractions should also be discussed. Processes such as these allow the student-athletes to be fully informed regarding their participation in athletics. Other preventative behavioral interventions may focus on team-building exercises, mental toughness, stress inoculation, and stress management.

According to some estimates, approximately 20 percent of athletic referrals present with strictly performance-related concerns, typically related to concentration issues, debilitating performance anxiety, or other stressors. Suinn (2005) developed a model of behavioral stress management that is applicable to athletics. On the practice fields, courts, or pools, Suinn noted that the most adaptive athletic responses are composed of physical and mental components, such as appropriate motor skills and preparatory physiological arousal, attention-concentration, and pairing cue recognition with appropriate responses. In addition, the athlete is attempting to transfer these components from practice to competition. Responses that must be extinguished include poor motor habits, reactions to extraneous stimuli, negative cognitions, and physiological arousal outside of the "optimal zone," while increasing the facilitative qualities of anxiety and reducing its incapacitating effects. Proper management of anxiety and stress includes removing or treating the stressful or anxiety-provoking stimuli, cognitive restructuring, modifying and extinguishing the maladaptive responses, or teaching the student-athlete to respond to new, more appropriate cues with accompanying responses that are appropriate and incompatible with maladaptive ones (for further information, see Suinn, 2005). Fortunately, certain types of assessment to test the effectiveness of these methods can be done in the therapy session, as well as while the athlete is in training, at practice, or at competition.

Athletics referrals not strictly related to performance issues primarily deal with academic or learning-disability evaluations as well as clinical concerns such as depression, anxiety, attention deficit disorder, injury recovery, eating disorders, substance abuse, and nonclinical concerns such as relationships, sexual orientation, and family-of-origin issues. Other than for academic and neuropsychological testing, which are governed by distinct guidelines, the use of empirically supported treatment approaches, including behavioral, cognitive-behavioral, stress-reduction, and interpersonal strategies, is typically indicated.

Anxiety

Many student-athletes, particularly those who compete in individual sports, initially present with concerns about "performance anxiety." They may report feeling anxiety during specific athletic situations or at certain venues due to previous poor performances at that event location. They may also report that they have difficulty focusing at the start of their athletic competition or have trouble sleeping before the big game or big meet. Further evaluation, however, often reveals a more pervasive pattern of anxiety that may include generalized anxiety disorder or social anxiety. In fact, a significant percentage of performance anxiety in student-athletes is a manifestation of more generalized anxiety disorder (GAD), and many athletes presenting with performance anxiety have comorbid major depression. Due to concerns about appearing "weak," athletes might initially minimize their anxiety-related stress.

With development of therapeutic rapport with team psychologists, athletes may be able to acknowledge the severity of their distress and acceptance of therapy for treating anxiety in important areas of their life outside of sports, including their approach to academics and personal relationships. Generally, anxiety disorders often develop in a predictable pattern. A student-athlete may experience or fear experiencing something negative in the context of either practice or competition; and every time that they encounter that feared situation, they choose to escape the anxiety by avoiding the stressful situation or by engaging in ritualistic behavior meant to allay that anxiety. These avoidance strategies or ritualistic behaviors eventually become problematic. Therapy often consists of 8 to 12 sessions that teach student-athletes to reevaluate the situations more rationally and to develop better strategies or behaviors for dealing more effectively with unavoidable circumstances.

Depression

Athletes often deny depression, perceiving it to be an admission of weakness. Instead, athletes often present with symptoms of insomnia, fatigue, weight loss, lack of interest in their sport, or even increased injury. Further clinical evaluation often reveals additional symptoms of depression. Indeed, depression is one of the most common of psychological ailments and is often comorbid with other serious psychiatric issues including anxiety disorders, substance abuse, personality disorders, eating disorders, and others. Athletes often feel depressed because of pressure from competing demands, feelings of being overwhelmed, or the consideration of major life changes such as retirement from their sport. Athletes who present with concerns about leaving their sport because they no longer enjoy it may actually be experiencing anhedonia (lack of interest in previously enjoyable activities) associated with depression. Educating athletes about depression symptoms and suggesting that they defer any decision about resigning from their sport until their depression has resolved are critical components of the initial meeting.

Subsequent therapeutic sessions should focus on resolving depressive symptoms through thought modification, as well as continued monitoring of the athlete's thoughts, feelings, and behaviors for other symptoms that may require psychopharmacological intervention or other medical assessment. One important element that may be overlooked is the possibility that the depressive symptoms may overlap with overtraining syndrome (see chapter 4). Recent evidence suggests that the same hypothalamic-pituitary-adrenocortical and sympthathetic-adrenal medullary axes may be disrupted in response to overtraining, as well as in major depressive disorders, warranting psychopharmacological intervention as well as psychotherapy. The former recommendation can usually be accomplished via referral to the team physicians.

As reviewed, student-athletes are not superhuman. They are similar to other college students who are completing similar psychosocial and physical developmental tasks; however, they are doing so in the context of also attempting to balance what could be considered two full-time jobs. Neither should student-athletes be regarded as exceptionally strong in the area of mental health. They may be at greater risk for developing psychological disorders, such as anxiety and depression, as well as for engaging in risky health behaviors when compared to nonathletes due to the intense pressures they face. Psychological problems may be newly emerging or may be a resurgence of preexisting emotional or behavioral issues. In summary, the need for support in the athletic population is great and should ideally begin with recruitment. Beginning at the time of signing would allow education of the prospective student-athletes and their families regarding typical pressures and problems they may experience while engaged in competitive sports at the university level, as well as inform them of available resources. The intervention approach proposed by the authors is a comprehensive model similar to the approach taken in developmental research "from the cradle to the grave" or from "recruitment to graduation."

We outline the elements of this model (MORE) here:

1. M: Mental Prep
   a. Proactive psycho-education of prospective student-athletes and their families regarding the common issues and problems faced by student-athletes at Division 1 level competition, as well as the nature of the relationship between athletics and team psychologists, emphasizing confidentiality and advocacy for student-athletes.
   b. Proactive psycho-educational seminars for coaches, coaching staff, sports medicine teams, nutritionists, and athletics department administrators.
   c. Stress inoculation and mental toughness training for athletes based on cognitive-behavioral programs.

2. O: Ongoing Check-in and Assessment
   a. Student-athletes, family members, and coaches are educated regarding signs or symptoms of potential problems for student-athletes which may require professional consultation.
   b. Team psychologists may send out e-health reminders to student-athletes and coaches regarding mental health hygiene and reminders about psychoeducational materials on important topics.

3. R: Referral
   a. Throughout Mental Prep and Ongoing Check-in & Assessment processes, student-athletes, their families, coaches, coaching staff, sports medicine staff, nutritionists, and athletics department administrators are reminded of the referral and initial clinical intake process, as well as the confidentiality of the process.

4. E: Evidence-Based Problem Solving and Treatment
   a. After initial clinical intake with team psychologists, an evidence-based problem-solving or treatment plan is developed which may include further assessment and testing (medical, neuropsychological, or clinical), biblio-therapy, or psychotherapy.

   b. Formulation of relevant clinical research questions to continue testing and modification of evidence-based treatment effectiveness.

CONCLUSION

Student-athletes are adolescents dealing with typical adolescent issues such as the developmental tasks and individual factors that impact a student-athlete's health, well-being, and performance, while living and working in what may be described as a crucible-like environment of pressures and relationships in which they are expected to perform. Many times, the pressures and relationships in the lives of student-athletes do not mesh well and may in fact be natural competitors. Because of this, student-athletes face an array of unique challenges. In this chapter, we reviewed the university environment in which many student-athletes live and work, the developmental factors that mitigate or exacerbate psychopathology, and briefly summarized psychological approaches for assessing and treating student-athletes. As pointed out by other researchers and clinicians, the mental health of student-athletes is most effectively protected and improved when an interdisciplinary team of caring professionals dedicated to the individual welfare of the student-athlete works together to meet these goals. These individuals include those in the departments of athletics/sports medicine (e.g., athletic trainers, team physicians, psychologists, and nutritionists), athletic academic affairs (e.g., academic advisors, deans, and professors) and people in the student-athlete's social support network (e.g., parents, teammates, romantic interests, and close friends).

REFERENCES

Arathoon, S. M., & Malouff, J. M. The effectiveness of a brief cognitive intervention to help athletes cope with competition loss. *Journal of Sports Behavior, 27*, 213–229.

Baum, A. (2006). Eating disorders in the male athlete. *Sports Med., 36*(1), 1–6.

Bennett, G. (2007). The role of a clinical psychologists in a Division I athletics program. *Journal of Clinical Sport Psychology. 1*, 261–269.

Birky, I. (2007). Counseling student athletes: Sport psychology as a specialization. In J. A. Lippincott, & R. B. Lippincott (Eds.), *Special populations in college counseling*. Alexandria, VA: American Counseling Association.

Broshek, D. K., & Freeman, J. R. (2005). Psychiatric and neuropsychological issues in sports medicine. *Clinics in Sports Medicine, 24*(3), 663–679.

Denny, K. G., & Steiner, H. (2008). External and internal factors influencing happiness in elite collegiate athletes. *Child Psychiatry Human Development, 40,* 55–72. DOI:10.1007/s10578-008-0111-z.

Etzel, E. F., Ferrante, A. P., & Pinkney, J. W. (Eds.). (2002). *Counseling college student athletes: Issues and interventions.* Morgantown, WV: Fitness Information Technology.

Etzel, E. F., & Watson, J. C. (2007). Ethical challenges for psychological consultations in intercollegiate athletics. *Journal of Clinical Sport Psychology, 1,* 304–317.

Flowers, R. (2007). Psychologist–sport psychologist liaison between counseling and psychological services and intercollegiate athletics. *Journal of Clinical Sport Psychology, 1,* 223–246.

Ford, J. A. (2007). Substance use among college athletes: A comparison based on sport/team affiliation. *Journal of American College Health, 55*(6), 367–373.

Gardner, F. L. (2007a). Introduction to the special issue: Clinical sport psychology in American intercollegiate athletics. *Journal of Clinical Sport Psychology, 1,* 207–209.

Gardner, F. L. (2007b). Clinical sport psychology in American intercollegiate athletics: Final thoughts. *Journal of Clinical Sport Psychology, 1,* 318–320.

Hack, B. (2007). The development and delivery of sport psychology services within a university sports medicine department. *Journal of Clinical Sport Psychology, 1,* 247–260.

Medic, N., Mack, D. E., Wilson, P. M., & Starles, J. L. The effects of athletic scholarships on motivation in sport. *Journal of Sport Behavior, 30*(3), 292–306.

Parham, W. D. (1993). The intercollegiate athlete: A 1990s profile. *Journal of Counseling Psychology, 21,* 411–429.

Perna, F. M., Antoni, M. H., Baum, A., Gordon, P., & Schneiderman, N. (2003). Cognitive behavioral stress management effects on injury and illness among competitive athletes: A randomized clinical trial. *Annals of Behavioral Medicine, 25*(1), 66–73.

Powell, D. H. (2004). Treating individuals with debilitating performance anxiety: An introduction. *Journal of Clinical Psychology, 60*(8), 801–808. DOI:10.1002/jclp.20038

Suinn, R. M. (2005). Behavioral intervention for stress management in sports. *International Journal of Stress Management, 12*(4), 343–362. DOI:10.1037/1072-5245.12.4.34

Watson, J. C., & Kissinger, D. B. (2007). Athletic participation and wellness: Implications for counseling college student-athletes. *Journal of College Counseling, 10,* 153–162.

Zillmer, E. A., & Gigli, R. W. (2007). Clinical sport psychology in intercollegiate athletics. *Journal of Clinical Sport Psychology, 1,* 210–222.

Chapter 9

The Female Athlete Triad

Sasha Steinlight and Margot Putukian

Exercise and participation in athletics promotes healthy lifestyle behaviors in girls and women. Exercise decreases the risk for diabetes, high blood pressure, and obesity. Young girls involved in sports have a lower risk for teen pregnancy (Sabo et al., 1999), substance use, and depression than their nonathletic peers. Female participation in athletics has been rapidly increasing over the last several decades. The involvement in athletics was enhanced by Title IX legislation, which was enacted in 1972 and stated that no one could be excluded from any educational program or activity receiving federal financial assistance based on sex. Basically, this meant equal opportunity for women to play organized sports. The result of this amendment was more girls and women joining athletic teams.

Title IX legislation eventually led way to the development of female athletics from the elementary, high school, and collegiate levels to the elite and professional level. More than 2 million girls participate in high school sports today as compared to several hundred thousand in 1972. There has been an approximately fourfold rise in the number of female collegiate athletes. New opportunities exist for female athletes to continue to participate in athletics after their college careers are completed, and these include the Women's National Basketball Association (WNBA), the Women's United Soccer Association (WUSA), and other professional female leagues. The existence of these leagues has encouraged young girls to join teams at an earlier age and allows girls to think and dream about participating in sports at a professional level.

While the increase in physical activity among females has been greatly beneficial to overall health, there is concern for those athletes who exercise to extremes. The "Female Athlete Triad" was first described in 1992 by the American College of Sports Medicine (ACSM) as the three components of amenorrhea, disordered eating, and osteoporosis. More recently, the triad has been redefined in 2007 by the ACSM to involve the interrelationship between energy availability, menstrual dysfunction, and bone mineral density. As new data has emerged, it has become clear that not all athletes have all components of the triad, but may display symptoms along a continuum of the disorders. Athletes and nonathletes of all levels are susceptible. Often symptoms are seen as part of a spectrum from health to disease, rather than following strict definitions.

Basic human metabolic function revolves around energy intake versus energy expenditure. Many athletic women are either unaware or ignore their daily energy requirements, leading to dysfunction of these systems. The energy intake of female athletes is often much less than the energy expended in their activities. This mismatch can lead to an "energy drain" phenomenon such that the energy intake is not enough to account for the energy output, and this can subsequently result in menstrual dysfunction.

Menstrual dysfunction in athletes occurs on a spectrum from eumenorrhea to amenorrhea. Emenorrhea is normal menstrual cycle function with menses occurring every 28 to 35 days, and approximately 12 menstrual cycles per year. Amenorrhea is absence of menstrual cycles for more than three months, and often less than 3 to 6 cycles per year. In the middle of the spectrum is oligomenorrhea, with irregular cycles and 9 to 12 cycles per year.

Bone density can range from normal bone health to osteopenia and, more severely, osteoporosis. Decreased bone mineral density is a risk factor for stress fractures as well as premature osteoporosis. Normal bone health depends on nutritional factors, estrogen levels, and activity level as well as genetic predisposition.

Eating disorders can also occur on a spectrum from experimentation with pathogenic behaviors to control weight to the most severe eating disorders of anorexia nervosa, bulimia nervosa, and eating disorders not otherwise specified.

In this chapter, the entities of the female athlete triad will be discussed in more detail. Essential in evaluating the athlete with components of the triad is an individualized approach, with early detection, and treatment essential in optimizing outcome and potentiating prevention. In working with athletes, families, and coaches, a multidisciplinary approach is often useful and helpful in optimizing care. This chapter will discuss strategies that the health care team can utilize to enhance the care provided to these athletes.

DISORDERED EATING

Eating disorders are biopsychosocial disorders that manifest as abnormal food behaviors. Disordered eating can be described by a constellation of behaviors. These behaviors include binging and/or purging, extreme calorie restriction, prolonged fasting or missed meals, preoccupation with food, distorted body image, fear of becoming fat, or use of diet pills or laxatives. Major eating disorders are classified as anorexia nervosa, bulimia nervosa, and eating disorders not otherwise specified. The *Diagnostic and Statistical Manual of Mental Disorders*, 4th edition (DSM-IV), written by the American Psychiatric Association, has defined eating disorders with guidelines for specific diagnoses. The criteria for diagnosis are outlined in Tables 9.1 through 9.3.

Table 9.1
Anorexia Nervosa

A. Refusal to maintain body weight at or above a minimally normal weight for age and height (e.g., weight loss leading to maintenance of body weight less than 85 percent of that expected; or failure to make expected weight gain during period of growth, leading to body weight less than 85 percent of that expected).
B. Intense fear of gaining weight or becoming fat, even though underweight.
C. Disturbance in the way in which one's body weight or shape is experienced, undue influence of body weight or shape on self-evaluation, or denial of the seriousness of the current low body weight.
D. In postmenarcheal females, amenorrhea, i.e., the absence of at least three consecutive menstrual cycles. (A woman is considered to have amenorrhea if her periods occur only following hormone, e.g., estrogen, administration.)

Specify type:
Restricting type: during the current episode of anorexia nervosa, the person has not regularly engaged in binge-eating or purging behavior (i.e., self-induced vomiting or the misuse of laxatives, diuretics or enemas)
Binge-eating/purging type: during the current episode of anorexia nervosa, the person has regularly engaged in binge-eating or purging behavior (i.e., self-induced vomiting or the misuse of laxatives, diuretics or enemas)

Source: Diagnostic and Statistical Manual of Mental Disorders (4th Ed., text rev.). Washington, DC: American Psychiatric Association, 2000.

Table 9.2
Bulimia Nervosa

A. Recurrent episodes of binge eating. An episode of binge eating is characterized by both of the following:
   1. Eating, in a discrete period of time (e.g., within any 2-hour period), an amount of food that is definitely larger than most people would eat during a similar period of time and under similar circumstances
   2. A sense of lack of control over eating during the episode (e.g., a feeling that one cannot stop eating or control what or how much one is eating)
B. Recurrent inappropriate compensatory behaviour in order to prevent weight gain, such as self-induced vomiting; misuse of laxatives, diuretics, enemas or other medications; fasting; or excessive exercise.
C. The binge eating and inappropriate compensatory behaviours both occur, on average, at least twice a week for three months.
D. Self-evaluation is unduly influenced by body shape and weight.
E. The disturbance does not occur exclusively during episodes of anorexia nervosa.

Specify type:
Purging type: during the current episode of bulimia nervosa, the person has regularly engaged in self-induced vomiting or the misuse of laxatives, diuretics or enemas
Nonpurging type: during the current episode of bulimia nervosa, the person has used other inappropriate compensatory behaviours, such as fasting or excessive exercise, but has not regularly engaged in self-induced vomiting or the misuse of laxatives, diuretics or enemas

---

Source: Diagnostic and Statistical Manual of Mental Disorders (4th Ed., text rev.) Washington, DC: American Psychiatric Association, 2000.

Anorexia nervosa is more common in females than males with a ratio of 10:1. The lifetime prevalence of anorexia is approximately 1 percent in females. Anorexia can result in severe morbidity and mortality such as electrolyte abnormalities, bradycardia or slowed heart rate, muscle and fat loss, low blood count, amenorrhea, osteoporosis, depression, suicide, and death. Bulimia nervosa occurs more frequently in late adolescents and young adults. Bulimia has a lifetime prevalence of 1 to 3.5 percent in the general population. A previous history of anorexia can be found in 30 to 80 percent of those with bulimia. Studies have shown up to 17 percent of college women engage in bulimic behavior. Women are often normal weight or slightly overweight, making it more difficult to diagnose. Bulimic behaviors have been found to be significantly more common in female athletes than the general population. Bulimia may lead to arrhythmias, electrolyte imbalances, gastrointestinal problems such as gastritis or constipation, or neurologic complications. Signs and symptoms associated with disordered eating can

Table 9.3
Eating Disorder Not Otherwise Specified

Eating disorder not otherwise specified includes disorders of eating that do not meet the criteria for any specific eating disorder.

A. For female patients, all of the criteria for anorexia nervosa are met except that the patient has regular menses.

B. All of the criteria for anorexia nervosa are met except that, despite significant weight loss, the patient's current weight is in the normal range.

C. All of the criteria for bulimia nervosa are met except that the binge eating and inappropriate compensatory mechanisms occur less than twice a week or for less than 3 months.

D. The patient has normal body weight and regularly uses inappropriate compensatory behavior after eating small amounts of food (e.g., self-induced vomiting after consuming two cookies).

E. Repeatedly chewing and spitting out, but not swallowing, large amounts of food.

Binge-eating disorder is recurrent episodes of binge eating in the absence if regular inappropriate compensatory behavior characteristic of bulimia nervosa.

Source: Diagnostic and Statistical Manual of Mental Disorders (4th Ed., text rev.) Washington, DC, American Psychiatric Association, 2000.

include irregular weight loss or rapid weight fluctuations, poor dental hygiene, discolored hands or scabs on knuckles, dizziness, unexpected electrolyte abnormalities, secretly eating, or drug and alcohol abuse. Some individuals may have a perfectionism attitude, a strong need to maintain a sense of control, have an obsession with their weight and appearance, or a decline in their performance. Most athletes will not meet DSM-IV criteria for eating disorders but will display behaviors from one or both disordered eating patterns. Disordered eating may manifest as low energy availability underlying other triad components.

Another entity, "athletic anorexia," has been described in athletes where the additional stressors of training, diet, and performance issues can cause an eating disorder to occur. These athletes often have a very intense fear of gaining weight or being fat though they are underweight (often > 5% less than expected). They often attain this low weight by energy restriction or excessive exercise. They can participate in binging, self-induced vomiting, and other pathogenic behaviors. In addition, they often have common psychological traits; high achievers, obsessive compulsive tendencies, perfectionism.

Eating disorders are a significant concern for high school and college athletes, and often very frustrating and difficult to treat. The complications of eating disorders are often significant, with a mortality rate of 6 to 18 percent, often due to overwhelming sepsis, cardiac arrhythmias, or suicide. Nutritional deficiencies are very common, and immune system dysfunction, electrolyte abnormalities, gastrointestinal disease, and low bone mineral density are also very common. The earlier that eating disorders are identified and treated, the more favorable the outcome.

Prevalence of the female athlete triad is unknown and varies widely depending on how each component is defined. Disordered eating has been seen in anywhere from 15 to 62 percent of female athletes. A large, well-controlled study that included DMS-IV criteria for eating disorders found a prevalence of 31 percent in elite athletes versus 5.5 percent in the general population. A second study with similar parameters found 25 percent of elite female athletes to have eating disorders as defined by DSM-IV criteria, whereas the same was true in only 9 percent of the general population. Sundgot-Borgen performed a study of elite female and male athletes versus controls designed to evaluate the prevalence of eating disorders in a variety of sports using self report survey followed by clinical interviews (Sundgot-Borgen & Torstveit, *CJSM* 14[1]: 2004). They demonstrated that 13.5 percent of athletes vs. 4.6 percent of controls had subclinical or clinical eating disorders. In male athletes, anti-gravitation sports were more often associated with eating disorders (22%), and in female athletes, those participating in aesthetic sports were most commonly associated with eating disorders (42%).

Internal and external factors increase the risk of disordered eating and the female athlete triad. Sports that require frequent weigh-ins may predispose an athlete to be more weight-conscious. Pressure to win and psychological pressures may lead to higher volumes of training. Societal pressures to be thin or look a certain way can affect an athlete's perception of what is considered normal. The media plays an important role in projecting thinness as equivalent to beautiful. Many professional athletes, models, and actresses are lean or emaciated, projecting an "ideal" physique. Magazines display slim cover models in swimsuits as a portrait of strength and beauty. Controlling parents or coaches may encourage weight loss in athletes or create an environment in which an athlete feels they need to control some aspect of their lives or training. Girls are starting sport-specific training at much earlier ages, creating a more competitive atmosphere in women's sports.

Disordered eating has a subset of risk factors including poor body image, a history of chronic dieting, low self-esteem and depression, family dysfunction including abuse, and biological factors. Cultural pressures including a historical emphasis on appearance create an environment of focus on a women's body. Thinness is often equated with attractiveness and social success. Some individuals believe their lives would be better if they were thin.

What puts athletes at risk for eating disorders? Often the same qualities that describe our most successful athletes are the same qualities that put athletes at risk for eating disorders. They often have high achievement expectations, are perfectionists, set goals, and are competitive, compulsive, and determined in all they do. This in association with other factors such as societal climate, family climate, biologic issues, response to victimization, self-esteem issues, role conflict, and lack of a sense of identity can increase the risk of eating disorders. In addition, athletes often feel that they are under pressure from coaches, parents, and judges to reach a low and often unrealistic body weight or body fat goal. The pressure to meet these weight goals can force the individual, who lacks knowledge of healthy behaviors, to resort to disordered eating behaviors. Athletes are often accustomed to, and willing to do whatever it takes to reach their goals. Though they may not be able to control how they perform, whether they start, or what others think, they can control what they put in their mouth.

Certain sports have been identified as carrying an increased risk of athletes developing the triad. This is seen in sports where performance is scored subjectively, such as dance, figure skating, and gymnastics. Endurance sports, distance running, and cycling emphasize low body weight. Swimming and diving, cheerleading, and volleyball all require body contour–revealing uniforms for competition. Prepubescent body habitus is frequently seen in elite-level gymnasts and is consistent with performance success. Wrestling, rowing, and some martial arts use weight categories for participation encouraging athletes to lose weight.

MENSTRUAL DYSFUNCTION

Menstrual dysfunction can present as oligomenorrhea, infrequent menses, or amenorrhea, absence of menses. Primary amenorrhea is defined as no menarche by 14 years old without secondary sexual characteristics, or 16 years old with normal development. Secondary amenorrhea results in a 3-month absence of menses after previously normal cycles, or a 12-month absence with previous oligomenorrhea. Menstrual irregularities in athletes are caused by low energy availability, resulting in decreased levels of estrogen. The body must maintain a normal energy balance in order for the reproductive system to function properly. An energy deficit reduces energy availability for cellular maintenance, thermoregulation, growth, locomotion, and reproduction. When energy is not available, the one function that is not necessary for survival is repro-duction, and thus this is often the first system to suffer consequences. The menstrual cycle is temporarily disrupted to preserve energy. This process is believed to begin at the level of the hypothalamus. Gonadotropin-releasing hormone, or GnRH, is released from the hypothalamus, signal-ing the anterior pituitary gland to release lutenizing hormone (LH). LH pulses from the pituitary cause a release in estrogen from the ovary. The disruption of the hypothalamic-pituitary-ovarian axis results in a func-tional hypothalamic amenorrhea. Higher levels of stress hormones, such as cortisol or growth hormone, have been observed in some cases.

The hormone leptin has been of particular interest recently. Leptin is a key hormone in regulation of appetite, metabolism, and the repro-ductive system. Secreted by adipocytes, leptin is a biomarker of body fat. Low leptin levels have been shown to correlate with infertility and may be seen in athletes with caloric deficits. Studies have shown that an increase in exercise alone does not affect LH secretion when caloric intake is appropriately increased to compensate for expendi-ture. Despite amenorrhea being a common occurrence in high-level female athletes, it is not a normal response to exercise and training. Menstrual dysfunction caused by hypoestrogenism may also result in adverse effects on bone mineral density, including an increased risk for stress fractures and early onset of osteopenia/osteoporosis.

Prevalence of amenorrhea in the general population is around 5 per-cent, whereas athletes range from 1 to 44 percent. Approximately 79 percent of athletes will have luteal phase dysfunction. Primary amenorrhea has been found in 22 percent of females in cheerleadering, diving, and gymnastics compared to less than 1 percent of the general population. Two small studies found secondary amenorrhea in 69 per-cent of dancers and 65 percent of long-distance runners, respectively. Data is variable based on patient demographics and definition of men-strual dysfunction. A larger study found secondary amenorrhea prevalent in only 2 to 5 percent of the general population.

OSTEOPENIA/OSTEOPOROSIS

Osteopenia is lower-than-normal bone mineral density. Osteoporosis is caused by low bone mineral density and disruption of the bony microarchitecture, resulting in an increase in bone fragility and risk of fracture. Low energy levels lead to a decrease in circulating estro-gen, which can then cause low bone mineral density and possibly osteoporosis. Low estrogen results in increased bone resorption, decreased calcium absorption, and decreased bone formation. Peak bone mass is achieved by 15 to 19 years of age in 60 to 70 percent of women. It is determined by genetic influence, hormonal factors, nutritional factors, and exercise and environmental factors. In the general population, bone loss begins around age 35. This process is accelerated after menopause due to decreased levels of circulating estrogen. In athletes, osteopenia mimics women who are postmenopausal or have premature ovarian failure or a pituitary tumor. Bone mineral density is best assessed by dual-energy X-ray absorptiometry (DEXA). The World Health Organization's (WHO) criterion for osteopenia is a T-score by DEXA scan of 1 to 2.5 standard deviations below the mean of a young healthy woman. Osteoporosis is greater than 2.5 standard deviations below the mean. T-scores are based on an average adult of the same gender and ethnicity. Z-scores, based on age, gender, and ethnicity, are more often utilized to evaluate premenopausal women and adolescents. The International Society for Clinical Densitometry (ISCD) states bone mineral density is lower than expected with a Z-score of 2 standard deviations below the mean.

Most athletes should have a bone mineral density 5 to 15 percent higher than nonathletes. However, it is not uncommon to find athletes with below-normal bone density. The ACSM states there is increased risk of osteoporosis if there is low bone mineral density based on Z-scores and the presence of secondary clinical risk factors such as chronic malnutrition, eating disorders, hypogonadism, glucocorticoid exposure, or a history of previous stress fractures. Current recommendations state bone mineral density should be evaluated every 1 to 2 years in athletes with a history of amenorrhea or previously documented osteopenia. Evaluation for bone loss should also occur after 6 months of amenorrhea or in athletes with a history of multiple stress fractures. Recovery from abnormal BMD may be slow. Recent studies have shown that bone loss is potentially irreversible. Early identification and treatment is critical to reducing future morbidity. A review of studies using WHO T-scores to determine bone mineral density found osteopenia in 22 to 50 percent of athletes and osteoporosis in 0 to 13 percent, compared to 12 percent and 2.3 percent in the general population, respectively.

DETECTION, EVALUATION, AND TREATMENT

Screening for female athlete triad should occur when an athlete presents to a physician's office. The pre-participation physical is an ideal opportunity to question the athlete on the various aspects of the triad. An example of a supplemental history that addresses issues specific to the female athlete can be found in Figure 9.1. In a Division I college, using a supplemental history for the female athlete, 65 percent reported irregular menstrual periods, and 30 percent reported that their menses had stopped completely at some time. In addition, 3.4 percent of athletes reported being diagnosed with an eating disorder by a physician, though 13.4 percent of athletes felt out of control of their eating patterns and 45.5 percent were unhappy with their weight. A variety of weight control methods were used to control weight; dieting/fasting (16.8%), diet pills (4.1%), excessive exercise (12.6%), vomiting (3.6%), laxatives (2.9%), and diuretics (0.3%). Finally, 16 percent of females in the survey reported a history of stress fracture confirmed by X-ray, MRI, or bone scan (Putukian, 2003). Evaluation can also be completed during annual health maintenance visits. Acute visits for injuries or stress fractures should prompt a physician to ask about eating habits and the menstrual cycle. If a female athlete presents with significant weight loss, signs or symptoms of disordered eating, amenorrhea, bradycardia, arrhythmia, or depression, a full screen of the triad should be performed.

When evaluating for disordered eating, some athletes may avoid straightforward questions about symptoms or avoid eye contact for fear of being identified. It is important to use a nonauthoritative, open approach to engage the patient in conversation. A detailed history should include questions about the individual's highest and lowest weight and ideal body weight. Ask about "forbidden" foods or controlling weight with excessive exercise, pills, or laxatives. Binging and purging behaviors or restrictive eating should be identified. Exercise patterns and training intensity for certain sports vary. A thorough exercise history and training schedule is important to determine if an individual is overtraining and may reveal body dysmorphic issues. Some athletes may do additional exercise outside of required training. History of multiple overuse injuries and stress fractures should be a red flag. A full menstrual history should be obtained, including age of menarche, frequency of menses, and the longest time period without menstruating. Some may experience physical signs of ovulation. Present or past use of hormonal therapy or any other medication or drug use should be documented. Early identification of athletes at risk may increase their rate of recovery or prevent injuries from occurring.

Other causes of weight loss, amenorrhea, and abnormal bone health should be ruled out prior to making the diagnosis of female athlete triad.

UNIVERSITY HEALTH SERVICES
SUPPLEMENTAL HISTORY FORM FOR THE FEMALE ATHLETE:

NAME: _____ Date of Birth _____ Class _____ Sport _____

1 How old were you when you had your first menstrual cycle? _____
2 How many days do you have menstrual bleeding?_____ What is the date of your last
   menstrual cycle?___
3 How may periods have you had in the past 12 months?   _____
4 Do you ever have cramping with your period?   Y   N
5 If yes, what do you do to lessen your symptoms?   _____
6 Have you ever had "irregular" cycles?   Y   N
   If yes, circle < 21 days or > 35 days between cycles?
7 Have you ever had heavy bleeding?   Y   N
8 Have you ever stopped having your period?   Y   N
   If yes, when and for how long? Give details (months/years).   _____
9 Have you ever had a stress fracture?   Y   N
   If yes, please list sites, dates, method of diagnosis (x-ray, bone scan, etc.) _____
10 Is there any family history of osteoporosis (thinning of bone)? _____
11 When was your last pelvic exam? _____ Last breast exam?_____
12 Have you ever had an ABNORMAL pelvic exam or PAP smear? _____
13 a. Are you currently taking oral contraceptives or hormones? Y / N
      If yes, why? (circle) birth control / irregular menses / no menses / painful menses / other
   b. Have you ever taken oral contraceptives or hormones? Y / N
      If yes, why? (circle) birth control / irregular menses / no menses / painful menses / other
14 Has a physician ever told you that you had anemia (low hematocrit or iron)? _____
15 What is your present weight? _____ Present height? _____
16 Are you happy with your present weight Y / N If not, what is your desired weight?_____
17 How many meals do you eat a day? _____ Do you take vitamins or
   supplements? _____
18 Highest weight: _____ Lowest weight: _____ Do you have trouble maintaining
   your optimal weight? Y / N
19 On an average in two days, how may servings of each do you eat? (Please circle.)
   Grains (cereal, bread, rice pasta)   0,1,2,3,4,>4   Fruits   0,1,2,3,4,>4
   Dairy products (milk, yogurt, cheese)   0,1,2,3,4,>4   Red meats   0,1,2,3,4,>4
   Beans, nuts, tofu   0,1,2,3,4,>4   Vegetables   0,1,2,3,4,>4
   Chicken, fish   0,1,2,3,4,>4   Eggs   0,1,2,3,4,>4
20 Do you ever feel out of control with your eating behaviors? Y / N
21 Have you ever tried to control your weight by: Dieting/fasting? Y / N Diet pills? Y / N
   Diuretics? Y / N   Vomiting? Y / N   Excessive Exercise? Y / N
22 Have you ever had an eating disorder? _____

Athlete Signature _____ Today's Date _____

(Princeton University Athletic Medicine 2009).

Figure 9.1.   Female triad supplemental history form.

A full workup including vital signs, height, weight, a complete physical exam, and pelvic examination should be performed. Laboratory studies such as urine pregnancy test, electrolytes, thyroid function tests, and a complete blood count may aid in diagnosis. An electrocardiogram (EKG) can identify arrhythmias commonly seen in disordered eating.

Studies have shown that a multidisciplinary approach to treatment has had the greatest success. This includes coaches and family members, a physician, a psychologist or psychiatrist, and a registered dietician. The valuable role that each individual plays increases the likelihood of success and sustained rate of recovery. An early and comprehensive intervention of disordered eating may also increase the rate of success. Psychological referral and treatment is the cornerstone of eating disorder treatment. It is important that the mental health provider is comfortable working with athletes and eating disorders, can understand the unique demands on student athletes, can provide a timely evaluation, and can, with permission, work as a team player in communicating with other members of the team. It is often helpful to have a "referral pattern" that can be followed when taking care of athletes with eating disorders. An example of a referral pattern that can be useful is shown in Figure 9.2. It is helpful for students, coaches, and others to understand the referral pattern with referral to a physician as a first step, and then referral to a psychologist. It is often helpful to have an "eating disorder policy" that helps athletes, coaches and parents understand the referral pattern as well as privacy issues. The eating disorder policy can also ensure that athletes and coaches know that weight control is not the responsibility of the coaching staff and weigh-ins should not be performed by coaches, but instead by health care providers (team physician, nutritionist, and athletic trainer) for medical reasons only. The athlete must have a desire to improve and agree with the parameters set by the team. Sometimes, an "athlete contract" is useful to ensure that an athlete understands the expectations of treatment as well as a lowest allowable weight under which participation is precluded. There should be a mutual agreement of the goal weight. Weight gain of 0.5 to 1 pound per week may be a reasonable goal. Exercise and training should be decreased by 10 to 20 percent. Training or competing may be continued if the athlete agrees to comply with all treatments, be closely monitored by health care professionals, make treatment a priority over training, and modify the training regimen.

The initial treatment for menstrual dysfunction is an interventional trial of increased energy intake. Ideally, this involves a nutritionist or dietitian familiar with athletes and the specific energy demands of

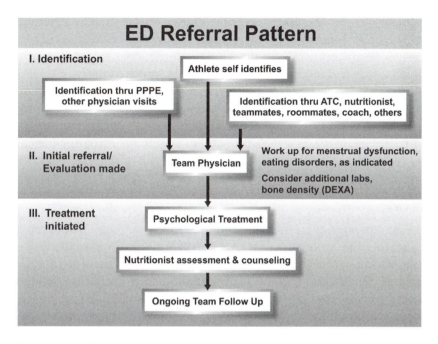

Figure 9.2. Disordered eating referral pattern.

the sports that they participate in. If the athlete is significantly under-weight, or has a history of multiple stress fractures and/or osteopenia or osteoporosis, a more aggressive approach may be necessary. Oral contraceptive pill (OCP), or hormonal therapy, has been used in the past for treatment of amenorrhea. This practice has been falling out of favor recently as it does not treat the underlying problem of energy imbalance and can "mask" energy deficit issues and bone health. The American Academy of Pediatrics states that hormonal therapy may be beneficial to mature amenorrheic athletes over the age of 16 or greater than 3 years post menarche. The ACSM recommends OCP use in athletes greater than 16 years of age in whom bone mineral density is decreasing despite adequate nutrition and body weight. Calcium 1,200 to 1,500 mg daily and vitamin D 400 to 800 IU daily sup-plementation is currently recommended for female athletes, especially those at risk for developing osteopenia. Bisphosphonates are not rec-ommended because of unproven efficacy in women of child-bearing age. They may also remain in bone for years, potentially causing harm to future fetus. Though the effects are limited, the use of nasal calcito-nin has been used for pre-menopausal women with osteoporosis with-out the concern for teratogenicity. The ultimate goal of treatment is to regulate menses and body weight with proper nutrition and training regimen. It is also important to consider the use of medications to treat the comorbid conditions of depression and anxiety, which can commonly occur and which should be treated appropriately.

Close follow-up with a physician will assist the athlete in achieving the agreed-upon goals. If not corrected, the triad may lead to long-term sequela. Eating disorders can lead to a significant increase in mortality. Menstrual dysfunction and osteoporosis increases the risk of hip and spine fractures.

PREVENTION

Prevention plays an important role in the female athlete triad. Educating the athletes, coaches, and staff about the female athlete triad may reduce the incidence of occurrence. It is important to educate the athletic training staff, coaching staff, conditioning staff, and physician staff on the signs and symptoms of eating disorders, as well as how to find help for an athlete at risk. Educating athletes on healthy eating and exercise regimens may reduce the risk of morbidities associated with energy deprivation. Coaches and athletic trainers should be aware of their athlete's behaviors and raise concern with the medical team early. Establish reasonable goals, set guidelines, and communicate with the athletes and staff. The athletic trainers should be prepared to enforce the guidelines set forth by the health care team. Develop a multidisciplinary team with mutual understanding and positive working relationships. Screen athletes when the opportunity presents itself. Early detection and treatment of disordered eating is important, and it is also important to dispel common myths about weight and nutrition. Athletes should be given sound nutritional advice regarding appropriate body weight and composition, and understand that "thinner is not always better," weight does not correlate to performance, and that performance can be impaired if nutritional intake is deficient. Through education, the hope is that some eating disorders and the sequela that can develop can be prevented. Finally, it is important to be aware, the triad is often underreported, unrecognized, and underdiagnosed.

RECOMMENDED READING

Beals KA, Meyer NL. Female athlete triad update. *Clin Sports Med*. Jan 2007; 26(1):69–89.

Bonci C, et al. National Athletic Trainers' Association position statement: preventing, detecting, and managing disordered eating in athletes. *J Athl Train*. Jan–Feb 2008; 43(1):80–108.

Costello L, Patel K. Eating disorders in athletes. In: *Netter's Sports Medicine*. Philadelphia: Saunders; 2009:184–188.

Frankovich R. The female athlete. In: *Netter's Sports Medicine*. Philadelphia: Saunders; 2009:72–85.

Hobart J, Smucker D. The female athlete triad. *American Family Physician*. June 2000; 61(11):3357–3364, 3367.

Nattiv A, et al. ACSM position stand on the female athlete triad. *Medicine & Science in Sports & Exercise*. 2007:1867–1882.

Nelson A, et al. Amenorrhea in adolescent athletes. *Pediatrics*. Aug 1989; 84 (2):394–395.

REFERENCE

Putukian M. Supplemental female history pre-participation survey; incidence of the entities of the female athlete triad. State College, PA: Penn State University; 2003.

Chapter 10

Concussion in Sport: Neuropsychological and Psychological Considerations

Ruben J. Echemendia

It is an almost daily occurrence that media outlets are reporting on professional, college, and high school players who have sustained concussions while playing sports. Some of these players recover fairly quickly, while others take longer to recover. The science underlying the assessment and management of sports concussion has expanded exponentially over the past 10 years. Indeed, the vast majority of what we know about sports concussions has emerged in the last 10 years. Similarly, the focus on concussion in sports as a significant injury that needs to be taken seriously has only emerged in the last several years. The goal of this chapter is to examine concussions from both neuropsychological and psychological perspectives to provide the reader with a up-to-date understanding of the injury, how it occurs, what to look for, how is it evaluated and treated, and when it is safe to return to play.

WHAT IS A CONCUSSION?

A cerebral concussion is a mild diffuse brain injury that is often referred to as a mild traumatic brain injury (MTBI). MTBI occurs as a result of a blow to the head or other part of the body, causing acceleration and deceleration of the brain inside the skull. Typically, players will report symptoms such as headache, nausea, vomiting, dizziness, balance problems, feeling "slowed down," fatigue, trouble sleeping, drowsiness, sensitivity to light or noise, loss of consciousness, blurred vision, difficulty remembering, and difficulty concentrating. Although there is no universal agreement on a definition of concussion, there does appear to be agreement on the clinical, pathologic, and biomechanical factors that are associated with MTBI. According to the most recent international consensus statement published by the Concussion in Sport group (Aubry et al., 2009) those factors are defined as follows:

> Concussion is defined as a complex pathophysiological process affecting the brain, induced by traumatic biomechanical forces. Several common features that incorporate clinical, pathologic and biomechanical injury constructs that may be utilized in defining the nature of a concussive head injury include:

> 1. Concussion may be caused either by a direct blow to the head, face, neck or elsewhere on the body with an impulsive force transmitted to the head.
> 2. Concussion typically results in the rapid onset of short-lived impairment of neurologic function that resolves spontaneously.
> 3. Concussion may result in neuropathological changes, but the acute clinical symptoms largely reflect a functional disturbance rather than a structural injury.
> 4. Concussion results in a graded set of clinical symptoms that may or may not involve loss of consciousness. Resolution of the clinical and cognitive symptoms typically follows a sequential course; however, it is important to note that, in a small percentage of cases, post-concussive symptoms may be prolonged.
> 5. No abnormality on standard structural neuroimaging studies is seen in concussion.

Athletes who sustain a concussive blow to the head often experience a state of confusion or disorientation that typically resolves within minutes. This initial state of confusion has historically been referred to as being "dinged." Unfortunately, the use of the term "ding" trivializes the importance and the severity of the injury (Guskiwicz, Bruce, Cantu et al., 2004). One of the most important aspects of this injury is that it progresses over time. In other words, the injury is an evolving one that is dynamic. Symptoms may occur immediately after injury, or they may take hours or days to emerge. It is not unusual for a player to initially report that they are feeling fine and then find themselves feeling sick on the bus or car ride home. The key point is to be vigilant for the emergence of symptoms over time and not to assume that a player who reports feeling well has not suffered a concussion. Although it is important for the medical team and coaches to recognize and eventually classify the concussive injury, it is equally important for the athlete to understand the signs and symptoms of concussion. More importantly, athletes must recognize the potential negative consequences of not reporting concussive symptoms, which include prolonged symptom recovery, the development of post-concussion syndrome, or even death. Once the athlete understands the injury, he or she can provide a more accurate report of factors associated with a concussion. Creating this awareness is of vital importance in the appropriate management of the injury.

WHAT ARE THE SYMPTOMS OF CONCUSSION?

Table 10.1 presents the most typical symptoms of concussion in a form that can be used to rate each symptom on a 0-to-6-point scale, which corresponds to mild, moderate, or severe classifications. This type of scale is typically used in concussion management and can be used to serially track both the absolute number of symptoms as well as the severity of those symptoms.

The symptoms contained in these checklists are not specific to concussion. In fact, they occur frequently within the general population for individuals who have not suffered a concussion. These symptoms can be seen in individuals who may have a physical illness (e.g., bad cold or flu), a psychological condition (e.g., depression, anxiety, ADHD), or even those who did not sleep well the night before. Consequently, obtaining a baseline symptom score is helpful to establish the type and frequency of any preexisting symptoms that arise from factors other than a concussion. Although very useful in assessing and managing concussive injuries, it is noteworthy that athletes are strongly motivated to return to play and may consciously or unconsciously minimize symptoms in order to return to the playing field. Stated bluntly, athletes lie about their symptoms.

Table 10.1
Concussion Symptom Checklist

Symptom	None				Mild	Moderate	Severe
Headache	0	1	2	3	4	5	6
"Pressure in head"	0	1	2	3	4	5	6
Neck Pain	0	1	2	3	4	5	6
Nausea or vomiting	0	1	2	3	4	5	6
Dizziness	0	1	2	3	4	5	6
Blurred vision	0	1	2	3	4	5	6
Balance problems	0	1	2	3	4	5	6
Sensitivity to light	0	1	2	3	4	5	6
Sensitivity to noise	0	1	2	3	4	5	6
Feeling slowed down	0	1	2	3	4	5	6
Feeling like "in a fog"	0	1	2	3	4	5	6
"Don't feel right"	0	1	2	3	4	5	6
Difficulty concentrating	0	1	2	3	4	5	6
Difficulty remembering	0	1	2	3	4	5	6
Fatigue or low energy	0	1	2	3	4	5	6
Confusion	0	1	2	3	4	5	6
Drowsiness	0	1	2	3	4	5	6
Trouble falling asleep	0	1	2	3	4	5	6
More emotional	0	1	2	3	4	5	6
Irritability	0	1	2	3	4	5	6
Sadness	0	1	2	3	4	5	6
Nervous or anxious	0	1	2	3	4	5	6

WHAT HAPPENS IN THE BRAIN?

One of the most difficult aspects of this injury is that it is largely invisible. Players who have sustained a concussion do not wear casts, slings, or orthopedic boots, or use crutches. Generally, they look "fine." Not only is this injury devoid of any external signs, it also does not appear on traditional neuroimaging techniques such as CT scans or MRIs. Instead of being a "structural" injury, concussions usually create a neurometabolic cascade that renders cells temporarily dysfunctional. These factors have created a fair amount of confusion for those trying to understand and manage this injury.

Typically, within minutes of a concussive injury, there are changes inside and outside of the cell membranes. There is an influx of calcium into the cells with a concomitant efflux of potassium that creates depolarization throughout the cells. The cells attempt to compensate by activating ion pumps, which increases the use of glucose (hyperglycolosis). Increases in lactate occur that have been associated with increased risk for secondary ischemic injury and possible predisposition for recurrent injury. As the metabolic cascade unfolds, the hyperglycolosis eventually creates a hypermetabolic state in which the brain is using vast amounts of resources to stabilize functioning. Unfortortunately, this hypermetabolic state is accompanied by disruptions in cerebral blood flow, which creates a mismatch between the brain's need for glucose and the glucose available due to restrictions in cerebral blood flow. A "hypometabolic" state then ensues that can last for several days after the initial injury. Decreased cerebral blood flow has been reported to last approximately 10 days following concussive injuries in animal models, which is consistent with the finding of an apparent 7-to-10-day period of increased susceptibility to recurrent injury. Eventually, cell functioning begins to stabilize and the metabolic crises resolves, returning to the cells to normal levels of functioning. This cellular process underscores the evolving and dynamic nature of concussions. In essence, a concussive injury is a process and not a static event.

HOW OFTEN DO CONCUSSIONS OCCUR?

Concussions in sport are a frequent occurrence, accounting for approximately 10 percent of all athletic injuries. The Centers for Disease Control estimate that 1.6 to 3.8 million sports-related concussions occur annually. These injuries occur across all contact sports, across all levels of play, and at all ages. In a study of ice hockey, lacrosse, and field hockey it was found that children aged 2 to 9 years sustained twice the proportion of head and face injures when compared to children aged 10 to 18. The NCAA Injury Surveillaence System published rates of concussion across a variety of collegiate sports. As can be seen in Table 10.2, concussions ranged from a low of 2.8 percent of game injuries in women's gymnastics to a high of 21.6 percent of game injuries in women's ice hockey. Concussions accounted for 6.8 percent of game injuries in football, 9 percent in men's ice hockey, and 4.8 percent of competition injuries in wrestling.

An interesting and fairly common finding is that women tend to sustain concussions at higher rates than men. For example,

Table 10.2
NCAA ISS 1988–1989 to 2003–2004

Sport	Percent of Game Injuries	Injury Rate per 1,000 Athlete Exposures	Injury Rank
Ice Hockey (W)*	21.6	2.72	1
Football (M)	6.8	2.34	3
Wrestling (W)	4.8	1.27	4
Ice Hockey (M)	9.0	1.47	2
Soccer (W)	8.6	1.42	3
Wrestling (W)	4.8	1.27	4
Soccer (M)	5.8	1.08	5
Lacrosse (W)	9.8	0.70	3
Field Hockey (W)	9.4	0.52	3
Basketball (W)	6.5	0.50	3
Basketball (M)	3.6	0.32	4
Gymnastics (W)	2.8	0.40	6
Softball (W)	6.0	0.25	3
Baseball (M)	3.3	0.19	5
Volleyball (W)	4.7	0.15	5

*Note: (W) = Women's; (M) = Men's. Source: Journal of Athletic Training, 2007.

concussions accounted for 5.8 percent of game injuries in men's soccer while accounting for 8.6 percent in women's soccer. Male basketball players sustained concussions at a rate of 3.6 percent during games, while concussions accounted for 6.5 percent of all game injuries in women's basketball. More alarmingly, male hockey players sustained concussions at the relatively high rate of 9 percent of game injuries, yet women hockey players had concussions at the rate of 21.6 percent of all game injuries. The difference between the rates of concussions in men and women is poorly understood although several factors have been implicated, including hormonal differences, differences in neck strength, differences in technique or differences in willingness to report concussion symptoms with the presumption that women are more willing to report symptoms than men.

Once an athlete has suffered a concussion, he or she is at risk for subsequent concussions. Studies have found that collegiate athletes are 3 times more likely to suffer a concussion if they had sustained 3 or more previous concussions in a 7-year period, and playing with 2 or more previous concussions required a longer time for total symptom resolution after subsequent injuries. Players also were at a 3 times higher risk for subsequent concussion in the same season. Repeat concussive injuries within the same season occurred within 10 days of the initial injury 92 percent of the time. Similarly, a study of high school athletes found that athletes with 3 or more prior concussions were at increased risk of experiencing loss of consciousness, anterograde amnesia, and confusion after subsequent concussion.

Although there is some evidence for the cumulative effects of concussion, several studies have found that self-reported concussion history is not related to decreased cognitive functioning. For example, we (Bruce & Echemendia, 2009) examined the relationship between concussion history and neuropsychological test performance on 3 different samples of athletes using traditional "paper and pencil" neuropsychological measures, a computer-based neuropsychological battery (ImPACT) and both ImPACT and traditional testing. We asked these college athletes to report on their history of concussions during preseason baseline testing and then compared those athletes who had no history of concussion with those who had one, two, and three or more concussions. No significant differences were found across concussion history groups irrespective of the type of neuropsychological test instrument used. We did caution, however, that these findings were based on relatively young athletes, and that it is quite possible that differences may emerge long term in these and other athletes.

In light of the contradictory findings that exist in the scientific literature, an individualized approach to concussion management appears to be most prudent, particularly since concussions are very heterogeneous and vary widely in symptom severity and resolution across individuals. Also of significance is the emergence of human and animal data that indicate that age may be an important consideration in the management of concussion. Younger athletes appear to have more severe symptoms that last longer than those of older athletes.

SIDELINE (ACUTE) EVALUATION OF CONCUSSION

A sideline or on-field clinical examination of players is critical for the identification and management of sports concussions. The primary goal of the on-field assessment is to identify any life-threatening conditions such as a developing intracranial bleed. If an athlete's symptoms are deteriorating, especially if there is deterioration to a stuporous, semicomatose, or comatose state of consciousness, the situation must be treated as a medical emergency, and emergency transport is required. If there is no deterioration in the athlete's condition, then a comprehensive sideline assessment should be conducted that includes a thorough history (including the number and severity of previous head injuries), observation of symptoms, player report of symptoms, a careful assessment of the player's recall of the events surrounding the injury, and specific tests of functional areas that are often disrupted following concussion, including simple tests of memory, concentration, motor coordination, and cranial nerve functioning. Simple questions such as, "What is the score?" "Who are we playing?" and "Who was involved in the last play?" help to establish the player's level of orientation. Certified athletic trainers (ATC) are in the best position to conduct these on-field evaluations by virtue of their training and experience. Unfortunately, many school districts and some colleges do not mandate the presence of ATCs at athletic competitions.

An emerging model in sports concussion assessment involves the use of brief screening tools to evaluate post-concussion signs and symptoms, cognitive functioning, and postural stability on the sidelines immediately after concussion. More sophisticated neuropsychological tests are then used to track recovery from the time of injury until the player is ready to return to sport. The results of neuropsychological tests, coupled with the physical examination and other aspects of the injury evaluation assist sports medicine professionals in making a safe and informed decision about return to play.

A recent addition to the sideline assessment armamentarium is the Sport Concussion Assessment Tool 2 (SCAT2) published by the Concussion in Sport Group noted earlier. The SCAT2 is a standardized method of evaluating athletes who have (or are suspected to have) sustained a concussion. It may be used with athletes who are 10 years of age and older. The SCAT2 contains the Glasgow Coma Scale, Standardized Assessment of Concussion (SAC, Cognitive Assessment), Maddocks Questions, a sideline assessment of balance and an examination of motor coordination. The SCAT2 has the advantage of being based on well-validated instruments and techniques, and is being used internationally.

POST-CONCUSSION ASSESSMENT

Comprehensive assessment of concussion is best accomplished within the context of a multidisciplinary sports medicine team that has access to a wide variety of assessment techniques. In addition to sideline assessment and medical evaluation, neuropsychological testing and assessment of postural stability are important tools. Although the use of neuropsychological assessment in sports is relatively new, neuropsychological techniques have been used to assess traumatic brain injury for many years. Neuropsychological testing in the assessment of MTBI involves the identification of a patient's functional and cognitive limitations as a result of the injury.

In order for a neuropsychologist to assess the presence of post-injury cognitive deficits, post-injury test scores must be compared with an estimate of pre-injury functioning. In contrast to most situations, athletes can be evaluated before sustaining an MTBI and the pre-injury scores can be compared to scores obtained post-injury. This "baseline" paradigm was first introduced by Dr. Jeff Barth and his colleagues at the University of Virginia. Using baseline testing with college football players, Barth et al. were able to demonstrate that neurocognitive deficits could be identified shortly after injury using a brief battery of neuropsychological tests. Recovery began shortly after injury with most athletes reporting complete recovery within 5 to 7 days post-injury. Several studies have now demonstrated that neuropsychological tests can identify neurocognitive deficits as early as two hours post injury with full recovery occurring within 5 to 10 days post injury depending on age and history of concussions. One study (Collins, Grindel & Lovell, 1999) examined college football players retrospectively and found that those athletes with a history of two or more concussions had poorer baseline performance on measures of information-processing speed and executive functioning when compared to the group of athletes with no history of concussion. An interesting finding was that athletes with a history of learning disability (self-reported) coupled with a history of multiple concussions had even poorer baseline performance than those athletes without a history of learning disabilities.

Another study (Echemendia et al., 2001) examined a multisport college population and found that a limited battery of neuropsychological measures can reliably differentiate athletes with concussion from uninjured controlled athletes as soon as two hours after injury. The concussed group of athletes scored significantly lower than control athletes two hours after injury and 48 hours after injury. Group differences were also evident at one week following injury. No differences were found between the groups at one month post injury. The results of this study were interesting because they revealed that athletes with concussions were unable to benefit from prior exposure to the test battery (practice effects) at the same level as the control athletes. This study underscored the dynamic nature of recovery following concussion since the neuropsychological performance of concussed athletes declined from two hours to 48 hours after injury, whereas the control athletes improved during this same time frame. More importantly, the neuropsychological test scores could statistically differentiate between athletes with and without concussion at 48 hours, whereas self-reported concussion symptoms as measured by the standard post-concussion symptom scale, could not distinguish between the two groups. This finding is noteworthy because it highlighted the limitations associated with relying exclusively on symptoms to determine return to play. The finding that somatic symptoms resolve prior to resolution of cognitive deficits has been demonstrated in several studies to date.

The SAC, a sideline cognitive screening instrument, was used concurrently with a set of traditional neuropsychological measures in a sample of college students (McCrae, Kelly, Randolph, et al. 2002). The SAC scores of athletes with concussion were significantly lower than baseline when compared with uninjured athletes. While SAC scores returned to baseline within 48 hours of injury, studies using more comprehensive neuropsychological measures showed typical recovery by 10 days after injury. These findings underscore the complementary nature of brief screening instruments and the more comprehensive neuropsychological batteries tests. Screening instruments such as the SAC appear to be useful on the sidelines and during the acute phase of recovery (initial 48 hours after injury), while neuropsychological test batteries appear to be more effective in identifying enduring neurocognitive deficits.

NEUROPSYCHOLOGICAL ASSESSMENT BATTERIES

As noted earlier, traditional neuropsychological test batteries consist of "paper and pencil" tests that are typically administered one on one. The development of computerized test batteries created a paradigm shift for neuropsychological assessment in sports. Four major computer-based batteries have been used in sports concussion management: ImPACT, CogSport, HeadMinder Concussion Resolution Index, and the Automated Neuropsychological Assessment Metrics Sports Medicine Battery (ANAM-SMB). These batteries allow for groups of athletes to be assessed using standardized, automated administration with immediate access to test results. Although each of these batteries is different in their composition and the number of functional domains that are assessed, each of these batteries allows for assessment of simple and complex information-processing speed, which has been shown to be a sensitive indicator of neurocognitive dysfunction post injury. These computerized batteries are much more cost-efficient than their paper-and-pencil counterparts and have extended the use of neuropsychological measurement pre and post injury to a much larger number of athletes when compared to the traditional batteries. However, they are not without their drawbacks: (1) They currently do not fully assess memory functioning because they are only capable of examining recognition memory; (2) they minimize the interaction between the athlete and the neuropsychologist, thereby reducing qualitative observations of performance; (3) effort and motivation are less effectively assessed and managed using group administration formats; and (4) they limit the ability to examine the process by which injured athletes solve problems and learn and remember information, which has been shown to be useful in the assessment of athletes with a concussion. These computer programs also introduce complex instrumentation error as scores may differ due to differences in timing accuracy across computer platforms, whether the test is administered via the Internet, the speed of the computer's processor, the type of mouse being used, etc. These sources of error are then multiplied each time that the battery is administered.

A substantial literature has emerged through the use of these computer-based programs. For example, a recent study used ImPACT to examine on-field predictors of neuropsychological functioning with a large sample of concussed high school and college athletes. At 3 days after injury, athletes with poor outcomes were 10 times more likely to have on-field retrograde amnesia and 4 times more likely to have reported on-field posttraumatic amnesia. No significant differences were found for loss of consciousness. A study using HeadMinder CRI found that cognitive impairment at initial postconcussion assessment (when compared with baseline levels) was a significant predictor of the duration of postconcussion symptoms. The findings of the Echemendia, et al., 2001 study were replicated by a subsequent study using the ANAM-SMB. In this sample differences between injured athletes and controls were not necessarily caused by poorer neuropsychological performance, but rather due to restricted or nonexistent practice effects in the concussed group when compared to the control group. Interestingly, this same pattern was observed when injured athletes with a history of concussions where compared to those with no history of concussions. Control subjects and athletes with no history of concussion revealed practice effects, while athletes with a history of previous concussions did not.

Although the field has some detractors (e.g., Randolph, McCrae, & Barr, 2005), there is generally a high degree of agreement that neuropsychological testing is an important part of the postconcussion evaluation process. However, some disagreement exists regarding the most appropriate timing and frequency of post-injury assessments. Initially, most research-based concussion surveillance programs evaluated players at specific intervals after a concussive injury. For example, athletes were assessed at 48 hours, 5 days, 10 days, and 30 days irrespective of whether they were symptomatic. This research approach is important when studying the natural course of recovery from concussion. Some have argued that this type of testing program unnecessarily exposes the athlete to multiple test administrations, thereby inflating practice effects. Their position rests on the premise that since players cannot be returned to play until they are symptom free, they should only be tested once their symptoms abate. There are good reasons for both of these perspectives. My perspective is that the number and timing of postconcussion assessments should be dictated by the question that the neuropsychologist is attempting to answer. If the question is, "Is this athlete ready to return to play?" then testing only once the player is symptom free, at rest and with exertion, is appropriate. However, if the question is, "How severe are this athlete's cognitive deficits?" then testing at several points post injury may be appropriate. This latter point is particularly important among youth athletes for whom academic accommodations may be needed.

We have discussed the use of traditional paper-and-pencil tests and the use of computerized test batteries. A "hybrid" model has developed where different combinations of paper-and-pencil and computer tests are used. For example, the Penn State Concussion Program has used a full paper and pencil battery and computer battery both at baseline and post-injury. In contrast, the National Hockey League and Princeton University use a hybrid model whereby computer-based testing is used at baseline with both computer-based tests and paper-and-pencil tests being used post injury. Since paper-and-pencil and computer-based tests have different strengths, the hybrid approach allows the neuropsychologist to capitalize on the best of both without the expense (financial and time) of administering full paper-and-pencil batteries at baseline.

An important consideration that has arisen is, "Who should administer and interpret neuropsychological tests?" The advent of computer-based programs has created widespread availability of these programs. The standard, automated administration and scoring aspects of these programs allows for easy access to individuals with limited amounts of training. Consequently, there is a very strong tendency for organizations to administer and interpret neuropsycho-logical test results without consultation with a qualified neuro-psychologist. The Concussion in Sport Group addressed this issue and stated, "Neuropsychologists are in the best position to interpret neuropsychological tests by virtue of their background and training." In a companion article, Echemendia, Herring, and Bailes (2009) examined this question at length and concluded, "The interpretation of neuropsychological tests requires comprehen-sive knowledge of the tests, their characteristics given a specific popu-lation (for example, team, sport), the athlete and his or her specific situation, psychological variables and many others. For these reasons we conclude that neuropsychological tests may be administered under the guidance of a neuropsychologist but that the interpre-tation of neuropsychological test data is best managed by a clinical neuropsychologist" (p. i35).

ASSESSING INJURY SEVERITY

Historically, the severity of concussions has been based on a series of "guidelines" that have been published by leaders in the field. Most of these guidelines were based on the presence or absence of loss of consciousness, the extent of memory disturbance (retrograde and post-traumatic), and symptom duration. In general, these guidelines were based on the clinical experience of the individual creating the guideline and not on the results of scientific investigations. The most widely used grading systems presented below had three grades of concussion: mild (I), moderate (II), and severe (III).

As can be seen in Table 10.3, these systems placed a great deal of emphasis on loss of consciousness (LOC) as an indicator of the most severe type of injury, irrespective of duration or the presence of other symptoms. The emphasis on LOC was based on the traumatic brain injury literature, where duration of coma was found to be a significant predictor of injury outcome. However, recent studies have cast doubt on this assumption, particularly in the case of sports concussion, where the period of altered consciousness is usually measured in seconds or minutes rather than hours and days. These studies suggest that while loss of consciousness may be related to greater early deficits, there is no significant relationship with overall injury severity or neuropsychological functioning.

Amnesia after MTBI has also been regarded as a marker of injury severity. Amnesia related to MTBI may take two forms: anterograde (or

Table 10.3
Concussion Grading Guidelines

System	Severity		
	Mild (I)	Moderate (II)	Severe (III)
Cantu	NO LOC PTA < 30 m	LOC < 5 min PTA > 30 < 24 hr	LOC ≥ 5 min PTA ≥ 24 hr
Colorado Med Society	Confusion NO LOC NO Amnesia	Confusion NO LOC Amnesia	LOC
American Academy of Neurology (AAN)	Confusion NO LOC Sxs < 15 m	Confusion NO LOC Sxs > 15 min	LOC

Note: LOC = loss of consciousness, PTA = Post-traumatic amnesia, Sxs = Symptoms.

post-traumatic) amnesia (inability to consolidate memory after the injury) and retrograde amnesia (inability to remember events prior to the injury). Both retrograde and anterograde amnesia are described by units of time. For example, the athlete had 2 hours of anterograde (post-traumatic amnesia) and 20 minutes of retrograde amnesia. In this case the athlete does not remember events within 2 hours after the injury and those that occurred 20 minutes or less prior to the injury. Research on amnesia has produced conflicting results; some studies find relationships between the presence of amnesia and neuropsychological test performance, while others do not. The weight of the evidence seems to suggest that LOC of less than a minute may not have significant post-injury sequela, whereas the presence of post-traumatic amnesia may be associated with poorer neurocognitive performance.

Cantu revised his grading system to incorporate the research on LOC, amnesia and symptom duration. His revised gudelines represent a move forward towards generating empirically based RTP criteria. He defined a grade I concussion as having no LOC or amnesia and postconcussion signs and symptoms (PCSS) lasting less than 30 minutes. A grade II concussion has LOC less that one minute, or amnesia and PCSS lasting more than 30 minutes. Grade III concussions have LOC in excess of one minute or amnesia for 24 hours or longer and PCSS in excess of 7 days. While Cantu's new system incorporates research findings on injury severity, very little empirical research speaks directly to the issue of *when* it is safe to return to competition and the consequences of being returned prematurely.

At present all concussion guidelines, with the exception of the Revised Cantu guidelines, grade concussion severity on the day of injury. A recent study of collegiate and professional athletes suggests that concussed athletes with symptom duration of greater than 7 days may have poor overall outcome, which provides support for the use of symptom duration as a factor in rating concussion severity. Consequently, it is important to monitor all postconcussion symptoms that the athlete may experience with final grading of concussion severity deferred until the symptoms have cleared. At present, most concussion management programs do not formally grade concussions. Several international consensus statements have recommended an individualized approach to concussion management and RTP.

RETURN TO PLAY

Presented in Table 10.4 are the RTP guidelines that accompanied each of the concussion grading systems described earlier.

The RTP guidelines differ on several important dimensions. The Cantu system required that a player be asymptomatic at rest and upon exertion for one week following MTBI, whereas the CMS and AAN guidelines allowed RTP to the same game if symptoms were absent for 20 minutes or less. At the other end of the spectrum, Cantu required one month and both the CMS and AAN required two weeks of no PCSS prior to RTP for Grade III concussions.

Table 10.4
Return-to-Play Guidelines

	Severity		
System	**Mild (I)**	**Moderate (II)**	**Severe (III)**
Cantu	RTP No Sxs 1 week (2) 2 weeks	RTP No Sxs 1 week (2) 2 weeks	Min 1 month 1 week no sx (2) Terminate
Colorado Med Society (CMS)	RTP if no sxs & no amnesia for 20 min	1 week No sxs	2 weeks No sxs
AAN	RTP if no MSE Changes or sxs at 15 min	1 week no sxs	2 weeks No sxs

Note: The Cantu system provides for additional conservatism if the player has had a previous concussion in the same season (2).

These guidelines served a useful purpose in the early days of concussion management, but there was much disagreement about which guidelines were the "best." There was no standardization of the use of the guidelines, and teams and programs varied widely with respect to which guidelines, if any, were being applied and whether they were being applied consistently. Many team physicians and athletic trainers felt that the guidelines were overly restrictive, particularly with college and professional athletes. It was also argued that "one-size-fits-all" guidelines were not appropriate for the management of a broad array of athletes.

Many clinicians believe that RTP guidelines are too conservative and, therefore, choose to make these decisions on clinical judgment of individual cases rather than on general recommendations. It has been reported that 30 percent of all high school and collegiate football players with concussions returned to competition on the same day of injury; the remaining 70 percent average 4 days of rest before returning to participation. Some RTP guidelines call for the athlete to be asymptomatic for at least 7 days before returning to participation after a grade I or grade II concussion. Although many clinicians deviate from these recommendations and are more liberal in making RTP decisions, recent studies provide some support for the 7-day waiting period to minimize the risk of recurrent injury. In one study athletes required an average of 7 days to fully recover after concussion. Same-season recurrent injuries typically take place within a short window of time, 7 to 10 days after the first concussion.

In contrast to the standardized "guideline" approach to RTP, Echemendia and Cantu (2006) proposed a descriptive model of the RTP decision. They characterized the return-to-play decision as a dynamic process involving the inclusion of many variables into relatively complex cost-benefit equations. Their model is depicted in Figure 10.1.

As can be seen, the model contains several major variable groups (factors). There are factors that are related to the concussion itself (Concussion Factors), factors associated with medical findings and history (Medical Factors), those that arise from the player (Player Factors), those related to the team (Team Factors), and any other extraneous factors such as field conditions, playing surface, quality and upkeep of equipment, facilities, etc. (Extraneous Factors). This model seeks only to describe the various elements of the RTP decision and does not proscribe a specific approach to RTP decision making, although it inherently endorses an individualized approach to the RTP decision. The model makes allowances for those elements or factors that have direct

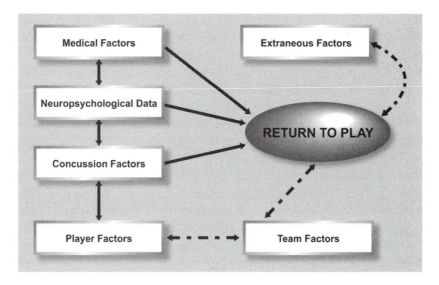

Figure 10.1. Interactions among return-to-play variables. (Adapted from Echemendia, 2006)

relationships to the RTP decision. For example, whether the player has positive radiologic findings, positive findings on physical examination, and the presence of physical symptoms has direct bearing on withholding the player from competition. Similarly, a decline in neuropsychological test scores relative to baseline has a very direct effect on the decision-making process. The player's history of concussions and the spacing of those concussions as well as the severity of the concussions have a direct and important impact on the RTP decision. To a lesser extent, the player's career aspirations, personality, style of play, family pressures, and their feelings regarding RTP are also considerations in the RTP decision. Although some would argue that team factors should not be a part of any RTP decision, in reality team factors are often considered in the RTP decision. For example, it is typical to evaluate whether the player is playing at a recreational level versus an elite or professional level, whether the player's position on the team is that of a journeyman or the "star" player, or whether the game or competition is relatively unimportant or whether it is the championship game. Other factors include whether the opposing team is known to be passive or very aggressive, and whether the player has been "marked" because their concussion history is known. Irrespective of how these factors are considered in the RTP decision, it must be underscored that athletes cannot return to play until they are symptom free at rest and upon exertion, and if available, neuropsychological test scores are judged to have returned to baseline levels. In other words, if the athlete is reporting concussion symptoms, it does not matter whether he or she is a professional athlete and they are playing the most important game of their life—the athlete should not play! It's simply not worth it.

One factor that was not included in the original model, but research has shown it should now be included, is player age. Recent data suggest that younger athletes may be more vulnerable to concussion, have more severe symptoms, and require a longer period of recovery when compared to older athletes. A related issue with younger players is the need for more frequent baseline neuropsychological testing. Since younger players' cognitive functioning continues along a developmental trajectory, baseline testing conducted when the child is 13 may not be representative of the child at 15 years of age. If the baseline neuropsychological data at a younger age cannot be assumed to represent the child's present neuropsychological "baseline," then the utility of the baseline data is questionable. It has long been recognized in psychological and neuropsychological assessment that age cohort norms must incorporate much narrower bands with children (e.g., 6 months) than with adults. In view of this, research must be conducted to determine the most appropriate interval for retesting children who are involved in high-risk sports. Until such research has been conducted, it is recommended from a practical standpoint that children 16 years or age and younger should have baselines renewed yearly.

Taken together, this model is highly consistent with the summary statements of Concussion in Sport Group since it calls for an individualized approach to RTP decision making that takes into account the complex and dynamic interactions that exist among variables. The model also strongly underscores the recommendation that RTP decisions cannot be based on one single test result.

It should be evident by now that the sports medicine team has an array of techniques and measurement instruments and can and should be used for the management of concussions. Although differences exist, several authors have arrived at a consensus that emphasizes an individualized, graded return to play following a return to baseline of postconcussion signs and symptoms. All signs and symptoms should be evaluated using a graded symptom scale or checklist when performing follow-up assessments and should be evaluated both at rest and after exertional maneuvers such as biking, jogging, sit-ups, and push-ups. Baseline measurements of neuropsychological and postural stability are strongly recommended for comparison with post injury measurements. Postural stability and neurocognitive functioning should return to baseline levels, given allowances for changes due to practice effects and measurement error. The need for cognitive rest in addition to physical rest has also been emphasized in the literature. In general, a progression of increasing physical and cognitive exertion occurs following a period of being asymptomatic (usually 24 hours). Once asymptomatic, the athlete may engage in light aerobic exercise, which is followed by sport-specific training during noncontact training drills. For the hockey player, this may include skating and shooting drills; the football player may participate in running drills or walking through plays, while the soccer player may engage in dribbling or shooting drills (but no heading). The sport-specific drills are then followed by controlled full-contact drills and ultimately unrestricted RTP. Progression from one level of exertion to the next is predicated on the absence of postconcussion signs and symptoms at the previous level. At no time before being released for full contact should the athlete be placed in a situation where he or she is at risk for a head injury. The amount of time spent at each level of activity may vary depending on player history of concussion or the duration of symptoms. For example, a player with a history of multiple concussions or particularly severe concussions can be held at a level of exertion or activity for 72 hours (or more), rather than just 24 hours. Conversely, individuals with relatively minor concussions may be progressed more rapidly, assuming that there are enough medical resources to appropriately assess injury severity. It is strongly recommended that consideration is given to more conservative management after recurrent injury, especially within-season repeat injuries. In these situations the athlete should be withheld from participation for an extended period of time after symptoms have resolved.

One of the most debated issues in concussion management involves return to play in the same day a concussion is diagnosed. As noted above, studies have found that 30 percent of all high school and collegiate football players with concussions returned to competition on the same day of injury. When symptoms resolve quickly (within 20 minutes) and the player remains asymptomatic following exertional activities, the question becomes whether or not he or she is at risk for another concussion or more severe catastrophic injury if returned to participation immediately. Some argue that an athlete should never be returned to the same game or contest if a concussion has been diagnosed. Others, typically elite college and professional sports, find this prohibition to be too restrictive. The Zurich Concussion in Sport Group discussed this issue extensively and concluded, "With adult athletes, in some settings, where there are team physicians experienced in concussion management and sufficient resources (e.g., access to neuropsychologists, consultants, neuroimaging, etc.), as well as access to immediate (i.e., sideline) neuro-cognitive assessment, RTP management may be more rapid ... There is [sic] data, however, demonstrating that, at the collegiate and high school level, athletes allowed to RTP on the same day may demonstrate NP deficits post-injury that may not be evident on the sidelines and are more likely to have delayed onset of symptoms" (pp. 188–189). Interestingly, at the time of this writing, the National Football League just recently announced a change in their concussion management policies that included more restrictive requirements for RTP in the same game. Taken together, several factors should be considered in making the same-day RTP decision, including the athlete's age and concussion history. If the athlete is 18 years of age or younger or has had a concussion, he or she should *not* be allowed to RTP in the same game or contest even if symptom free at rest and on exertion. He or she should be held out of play for at least 24 hours. If the adult athlete undergoes a comprehensive examination by a well-qualified professional and is returned to play in the same game, he or she must be monitored closely for the next 48 to 72 hours to assess for delayed onset of symptoms. However, any athlete who experiences loss of consciousness or amnesia should be disqualified from participating on the day of injury.

HOW MANY IS TOO MANY?

There are no prospective studies that provide guidance on when an athlete's season or career should be terminated. Although not empirically based, many clinicians believe that 3 mild concussions in one season should terminate participation in that season. Similarly, some believe that 2 moderate or severe concussions should terminate the season. Although empirically derived recommendations cannot be made, clinical experience suggests that terminating a player's season because of multiple concussions is warranted. If the season is terminated, it is recommended that a sufficient amount of time (for example, 3 months) with the player free of symptoms at rest and following exertion should elapse before returning to play. Retirement from contact or collision sports participation should be seriously considered if the player's neurologic examination has not returned to normal or if any postconcussion signs or symptoms are present at rest or during exertion. Additional criteria that may preclude return to competition include persistent abnormal findings on neuropsychological test batteries or failure to return to baseline on neuropsychological tests, and the presence of a lesion on imaging studies that places the athlete at increased risk of further injury.

Two key factors in determining when a player should be encouraged to retire from contact or collision sports are symptom duration and the force of the blow that is needed to cause a concussion. If the duration of postconcussion symptoms progressively increases with subsequent concussions, or if postconcussion symptoms last 3 months or longer in a player with multiple concussions, retirement from sport should be considered. The force of a blow needed to produce a concussion is also used to determine whether or not a player should consider retirement. If mild, indirect blows where the head is not struck directly or relatively mild hits to the head produce prolonged postconcussion symptoms, then retirement should be considered. This is particularly true if a pattern becomes evident where lesser and lesser blows produce a greater number of symptoms that are more intense and have prolonged duration.

The long-term consequences of repeated concussions have also been widely discussed, and there is a pronounced absence of longitudinal prospective studies. However, recent studies strongly indicate that this is an area that requires significant in-depth study with well designed, well-controlled prospective methodologies. Of interest are survey data gathered by Guskiewicz and his colleagues (2005), who asked retired professional football players about their history of concussion, psychological symptoms, and cognitive symptoms. Using these self-report data, it was found that athletes with 3 or more reported concussions had a fivefold prevalence of mild cognitive impairment. Additionally, retired players with 3 or more concussions had a threefold prevalence of self-reported significant memory problems in comparison with retirees who did not have a history of concussion. Although these self-report data must be viewed with caution, they do suggest that attention must be focused on this issue. In a related study, Guskiewicz and his colleagues found a relationship between self-reported recurrent concussion and self-reported clinical depression among retired professional football players. These findings, coupled with recent autopsy evidence of chronic traumatic encephalopathy among professional athletes with a history of repeated concussions, sound an important alarm for the study of long-term consequences of concussions.

PSYCHOLOGICAL CONSIDERATIONS IN MTBI

Psychological factors in MTBI may occur from direct effects of the brain injury as well as effects that are secondary or indirectly related to the injury. Direct effects are those that arise from the injury itself and typically involve a set of behavioral symptoms, including anxiety, depression, irritability, emotional lability, and changes in personality functioning. Like most symptoms associated with MTBI, these symptoms are typically self-limiting and resolve within a relatively short time frame (e.g., 5 to 10 days). However, in a small number of athletes, these symptoms may last for an extended period of time and develop into postconcussion syndrome. Athletes who experience these symptoms for a protracted period of time (e.g., greater than 2 weeks) should be referred to a mental health professional who is well versed in the signs and symptoms of sport-related concussion.

Indirect psychological effects arise from a variety of sources. MTBI was described earlier as an "invisible" injury since there are no outward signs of the injury. Players who are held out of competition due to concussion symptoms often become anxious or depressed because they feel the pressure to compete from their colleagues, coaches, parents, and friends because they look "fine." They fear that they are being judged as "weak" or "soft" for not playing. Certainly no one would question the toughness of an athlete who is not playing with a cast or with an obvious limp. Similarly, the athletic culture of playing through pain encourages athletes to downplay or deny their symptoms. Players who report their symptoms accurately may also been seen as "soft." These factors often interact such that the player begins to question his or her own "toughness" and willingness to play.

Players who sustain a concussion are often frightened or bewildered by the experience. They do not understand their symptoms and typically do not know how long the symptoms will last. In fact, many athletes experience the symptoms but fail to recognize that they have sustained a concussion. As noted above, athletes who sustain a concussion are typically told to rest, both physically and cognitively. At times, athletes become depressed not from the direct effects of the concussion, but rather from the fact that they are no longer as physically active as they were before and are concerned about losing their spot on the team and becoming physically deconditioned. If they are in school or college, these athletes may have a very difficult time focusing their concentration during class, feel less capable of learning and remembering information, fatigue easily, and experience symptom exacerbation with focused attention (e.g., sitting in class, studying), among others. These factors then serve to exacerbate feelings of both depression and anxiety. It is important for the sports medicine team to intervene early on several fronts: (1) reassure the athlete that these symptoms are typically time-limited and will improve over time; (2) provide the athlete with information regarding the symptoms of concussion (i.e., the types of symptoms and their dynamic nature); (3) make environmental modifications such as requesting scholastic accommodations; and (4) direct intervention with anxiety and depression such as cognitive behavior therapy and relaxation techniques.

CONCLUSIONS

Cerebral concussions are a common occurrence across a broad range of sports, ages, and levels of play. Although concussions were viewed historically as a nuisance injury that was often brushed aside or ridiculed, we now know that concussions can be a significant injury that must be taken seriously. We have an emerging science that has (1) been able to identify the signs and symptoms of concussion, (2) described the pathophysiology of the injury, and (3) developed measurement techniques to more objectively assess the sequela of the injury. Neuropsychology and psychology have had important roles in the development of this science and will continue to do so in the future. While there are many aspects of concussions that we still do not fully understand, and while there is a lack of consensus among experts in the area on certain issues, there is one area in which there is clear and consistent advice: Players should not be allowed to return to play until they are symptom free at rest and on exertion, and they have returned to their neurocognitive baseline. We need to move forward with our research to answer important questions such as the long-term psychological and neurological consequences of repeated concussion and to develop prevention-oriented strategies. Most importantly, we need to educate athletes, their families, coaches, physicians, and policy makers to recognize and appropriately manage this injury. In doing so, we will enhance player safety while allowing athletes to engage in the sports that they love.

RECOMMENDED READING

Echemendia, R. J. (Ed.) (2006). *Sports neuropsychology: Assessment and management of traumatic brain injury.* New York: Guilford Press.

Lovell, M., Echemendia, R., Barth, J., & Collins, M. (Eds.) (2004). *Traumatic brain injury in sports: An international neuropsychological perspective.* Lisse: Swets & Zeitlinger.

McCrory, P., Meeuwisse, W., Johnston, K., Dvorak, J., Aubry, M., Molloy, M. and Cantu, R. (2009). Consensus Statement on Concussion in Sport 3rd International Conference on Concussion in Sport held in Zurich, November 2008. *Clinical Journal of Sports Medicine, 19,* 185–195.

Moser, R. S., Iverson, G. L., Echemendia, R. J., Lovell, M./R., Schatz, P., Webbe, F., Ruff, R. & Barth, J. T. (2007). Neuropsychological evaluation in the diagnosis and management of sports-related concussion. *Archives of Clinical Neuropsychology, 22,* 909–916.

REFERENCES

Barth, J. T., Alves, W., Ryan, T., Macciocchi, S., Rimel, R. W., Jane, J. J., et al. (1989). Mild head injury in sports: Neuropsychological sequelae and recovery of function. In H. Levin, J. Eisenberg, & A. Benton (Eds.), *Mild head injury* (pp. 257–275). New York: Oxford University Press.

Bruce, J. & Echemendia, R. J. (2009). History of multiple concussions is not associated with reduced cognitive abilities. *Neurosurgery, 64*(1), 100–106.

Collins, M., Grindel, S., & Lovell, M. (1999). Relationship between concussion and neuropsychological performance in college football players. *Journal of the American Medical Association, 282,* 964–970.

Echemendia, R. J., Herring, S., & Bailes, J. (2009). Who should administer and interpret neuropsychological tests? *British Journal of Sports Medicine, 43,* 32–35.

Echemendia, R. J., Putukian, M., Mackin, S., Julian, L., & Shoss, N. (2001). Neuropsychological test performance prior to and following sports-related mild traumatic brain injury. *Clinical Journal of Sport Medicine, 11,* 23–31.

Guskiewicz, K., Bruce, S., Cantu, R., et al. (2004). National Athletic Trainer's position statement: Management of sport-related concussion. *Journal of Athletic Training, 39,* 280–297.

Guskiewicz, K. M., Marshall, S. W., Bailes, J. et al. (2005). Association between recurrent concussion and late-life cognitive impairment in professional football players. *Neurosurgery, 57,* 719–726.

Journal of Athletic Training (2007). 42(2).

McCrory, P., Meeuwisse, W., Johnston, K., Dvorak, J., Aubry, M., Molloy, M., & Cantu, R. (2009). Consensus statement on concussion in sport 3rd International Conference on Concussion in Sport held in Zurich, November 2008. *Clinical Journal of Sports Medicine, 19,* 185–195.

Randolph, C., McCrae, M., & Barr, W. (2005). Is neuropsychological testing useful in the medical management of sport-related concussion?. *Journal of Athletic Training, 40,* 136–151.

Index

About the Editors and Contributors

EDITORS

Ruben J. Echemendia, PhD, is a clinical neuropsychologist. He is the Director of the National Hockey League's Neuropsychological Testing Program, Chair of the NHL's Concussion Working Group, the consulting clinical neuropsychologist to the U.S. Soccer National Teams, founder of the Penn State University Concussion Program, and serves as a consultant to numerous recreational, high school, college and professional sports teams. He serves on the U.S. Lacrosse Sports Science and Safety Committee and the U.S. Soccer Medical Advisory Committee. Dr. Echemendia has recently become the Chair of Major League Soccer's Concussion Group. Dr. Echemendia has had extensive clinical and research experience with sports-related concussions and has spoken internationally on issues related to traumatic brain injury in sports. He is currently in independent practice after having spent 18 years on the faculty of Penn State University. He is a Past President of the National Academy of Neuropsychology and a Fellow of both the National Academy of Neuropsychology and the American Psychological Association. He has published widely and has been a featured guest on several television and radio programs.

Claude T. Moorman III, MD, a board-certified orthopedic surgeon, is the Director of Duke Sports Medicine and head team physician for Duke University athletics. He attended the University of Cincinnati Medical School and was a resident in orthopedic surgery at Duke University

Medical Center with fellowship training in sports medicine at the Hospital for Special Surgery in New York City.

CONTRIBUTORS

Donna K. Broshek, PhD, is a clinical neuropsychologist and Associate Professor of Psychiatry & Neurobehavioral Sciences at the University of Virginia (UVA) School of Medicine. She is Co-Director of the Neurocognitive Assessment Laboratory and Associate Director of the Brain Injury and Sports Concussion Institute. She is Director of the Medical Psychology Fellowship Program and a psychological consultant to the UVA Athletics Department. Dr. Broshek is a Fellow of the National Academy of Neuropsychology.

Bruce Burke is the founder of Fitness Consultants Inc. in State College, Pennsylvania. Through his personal fitness training business, One on One, he has worked with thousands of individuals over the last 24 years. This experience has given him a unique insight into not only the psychological challenges people face as they consider becoming fit, but the practical challenges as well.

Kym Burke is the co-owner of Fitness Consultants Inc. in State College, Pennsylvania. Through her personal fitness training business, One on One, she has worked with thousands of individuals over the last 24 years. This experience has given her a unique insight into not only the psychological challenges people face as they consider becoming fit, but the practical challenges as well.

Katherine E. Cutitta is a practicum student in the Neurocognitive Assessment Laboratory at the University of Virginia School of Medicine and has been active in several research projects targeting improving adherence in HIV patients from rural and underserved populations. She is completing her psychology degree from Virginia Polytechnic Institute and she is the past president of an organization of scholar athletes dedicated to sportsmanship.

Jason R. Freeman, PhD, is a clinical neuropsychologist and Associate Professor of Psychiatry & Neurobehavioral Sciences at the University of Virginia (UVA) School of Medicine and Associate Director of the Brain Injury and Sports Concussion Institute. He is a psychological consultant to the UVA Athletics Department and UVA Ryan White HIV Clinic. Dr. Freeman is also a neuropsychological consultant to the UVA abdominal transplant teams.

Christopher M. Janelle, PhD, is Associate Professor and Director of the Performance Psychology Laboratory in the Department of Applied Physiology and Kinesiology at the University of Florida. His research interests focus on the interactive nature of emotion, attention, and movement as related to human performance and health issues, and he is currently funded by the National Institute of Mental Health (NIMH) and the American Heart Association (AHA) for his work in these areas. He has published over 50 scientific articles and book chapters, and has made over 65 presentations worldwide dealing with these topics. He also coauthored the *Handbook of Sport Psychology* (2001). Dr. Janelle was awarded the 2002 Dorothy Harris Memorial Award for early career excellence by the Association for the Advancement of Applied Sport Psychology (AAASP). He reviews papers for the leading journals in the field, is section editor for the *International Journal of Sport and Exercise Psychology* and *Research Quarterly for Exercise and Sport*, and sits on four editorial boards, including the *Journal of Sport & Exercise Psychology* and the newly formed *International Review of Sport and Exercise Psychology*. In addition to his scholarly work, Dr. Janelle has worked as a sport psychology consultant with collegiate, Olympic, professional, and youth sport athletes.

Göran Kenttä earned his PhD in psychology at Stockholm University in 2001. Dr. Kenttä currently holds a research position at the Swedish School of Sport and Health Sciences. He is also the past president of the Swedish sport psychological association. The majority of research and publications has focused on elite-level athletes and the training process with a stress-recovery perspective. He is currently involved with the Swedish Olympic Committee and the Swedish National Sport Federation (NGB) in order to develop strategies for sport psychological support for the elite athletes and coaches.

Derek T. Y. Mann, PhD, is a Performance Enhancement Consultant and cofounder of the Performance Psychology Group, LLC (PPG), an organization responsible for providing coaching services to athletes and corporate executives throughout North America. Dr. Mann has spent several years investigating the impact of emotion on human performance with elite populations. His work has been published in the *Journal of Sport and Exercise Psychology*, the *Sport Psychologist*, and the *Journal of Human Movement Studies*. He has also served as a contributing editor to several leading academic and professional journals. Dr. Mann currently holds the position of Senior Research Associate at Multi-Health Systems, where he has contributed to the growth and accessibility of Emotional Intelligence through assessment, training and development, and professional presentations throughout North America.

Susana Quintana Marikle earned her master's degree in mental health counseling from the University of Central Florida and her bachelor's degree in psychology from Florida Atlantic University. She is currently a clinical psychology doctoral student at Nova Southeastern University within the Center for Psychological Studies and expects to receive her PsyD in 2012. Ms. Quintana Marikle is an active member of the NSU Sport Psychology research team and presently serves as the team's research coordinator. She has published articles on the mental health benefits of exercise and her research interests include sport-related concussion as well as applied sport psychology.

Margot Putukian, MD, is the Director of Athletic Medicine and Head Team Physician at Princeton Univeristy. She received her B.S. degree in biology from Yale University, then completed her internship and residency in Primary Care Internal Medicine at Strong Memorial Hospital in Rochester, New York. She completed her fellowship in sports medicine at Michigan State University, in East Lansing. Dr. Putukian is a charter member of the American Medical Society for Sports Medicine (AMSSM), where she served as President during 2004–2005, and is currently President-elect of the AMSSM Foundation Board. She is also currently on the Board of Trustees for the American College of Sports Medicine. She has served on the NCAA Competitive Safeguards and Medical Aspects of Sports Committee, and is currently the Chair for the U.S. Lacrosse Sports Science & Safety Committee. Dr. Putukian is also a team physician for U.S. Soccer and U.S. Lacrosse.

Kristy Quackenbush is completing her clinical psychology graduate training and is aiming for a career at a university counseling center with the main responsibility of counseling student-athletes.

John S. Raglin, PhD, FACSM, is currently a professor and director of graduate studies in the Department of Kinesiology at Indiana University in Bloomington. His research interests include examining the efficacy of exercise to enhance mental health, the influence of emotion and personality, and the psychobiological consequences of intense athletic training. He is a fellow in the American Psychological

Association, American College of Sports Medicine and the American Academy of Kinesiology and Physical Education.

Stephen A. Russo, PhD, has worked as an applied sport psychologist since 1998, serving as the Director of Sport Psychology at two world-class training facilities. He is the former director of Sport Psychology at the University of Pittsburgh Medical Center (UPMC)–Center for Sports Medicine and was also the staff Sport Psychologist at the International Junior Golf Academy (IJGA) in Hilton Head, South Carolina. In these roles, Dr. Russo served as a sport consultant to numerous professional athletes, coaches, organizations, and university athletic departments. He is a licensed clinical psychologist and an active member of both the Association for Applied Sport Psychology and the Sport & Exercise Division of the American Psychological Association (Div. 47). Currently, Dr. Russo serves as an Assistant Professor within the Center for Psychological Studies at Nova Southeastern University in Fort Lauderdale, Florida. He also works as the Director of Sport Psychology for the NSU Athletic Department and the Sport Medicine Clinic within the NSU College of Osteopathic Medicine. In this capacity he serves as a member of a multidisciplinary sports medicine team, comprised of professionals from the areas of physical therapy, athletic training, nutrition, and osteopathic medicine.

Christine M. Salinas is completing a predoctoral clinical psychology internship at Emory University Medical Center in Atlanta, Georgia, and aims for a career in pediatric clinical neuropsychology.

Sasha Steinlight, MD, is currently a sports medicine fellow at UMDNJ–Robert Wood Johnson Medical School. She assists the team physicians at Rutgers University and Princeton University. She received her undergraduate degree from Indiana University in Bloomington, Indiana, earning a B.S. in biochemistry. Dr. Steinlight then attended UMDNJ–New Jersey Medical School where she earned her MD. She was a member of AOA honor society. After medical school, she completed her residency in family medicine at the University of Pennsylvania in Philadelphia

Stephanie J. Tiedemann is completing her clinical psychology graduate training and is aiming for a career in sports and health psychology at a medical facility.

Desi Alonzo Vásquez Guerrero, PhD, is a Fellow in the Department of Psychiatry and Neurobehavioral Sciences at the University of

Virginia Health System. He currently treats student-athletes at the UVA Brain Injury and Sports Concussion Institute and Neurocognitive Assessment Laboratory. In 2009, he was awarded the *Young Scientist Award* by the University of Virginia Housestaff Council for excellence in scientific merit while engaging in clinical research.

Ralph A. Vernacchia, PhD, is a professor of physical education at Western Washington University where he coordinates the undergraduate and graduate sport psychology programs. He is the director of the WWU Center for Performance Excellence and is a fellow and certified consultant of the Association for Applied Sport Psychology.

Frank M. Webbe, PhD, is a professor of psychology at Florida Institute of Technology. He is a former president of the Division of Exercise and Sport Psychology of the American Psychological Association and a Fellow of that Association. He has written widely on sport psychology and sport neuropsychology.